Autistic Spectrum Disorders in the Early Years

Autistic Spectrum Disorders in the Early Years

Lynn Plimley, Maggie Bowen
and Hugh Morgan

Paul Chapman
Publishing

First published 2007

Paul Chapman Publishing
A SAGE Publications Company
1 Oliver's Yard
55 City Road
London EC1Y 1SP

SAGE Publications Inc
2455 Teller Road
Thousand Oaks, California 91320

SAGE Publications India Pvt Ltd
B 1/I 1 Mohan Cooperative Industrial Area
Mathura Road, Post Bag 7
New Delhi 110 044

Library of Congress Control Number: 2006932497

A catalogue record for this book is available from the
British Library

ISBN-1-4129-2314-X   ISBN-978-1-4129-2314-9
ISBN-1-4129-2315-8   ISBN-978-1-4129-2315-6 (pbk)

Typeset by C&M Digitals (P) Ltd., Chennai, India
Printed in Great Britain by Cromwell Press Ltd, Trowbridge, Wiltshire
Printed on paper from sustainable resources

Contents

Lynn Plimley

Lynn Plimley trained to teach children with special educational needs in the mid-70s, and has worked with children with ASD since 1979.

She has worked in generic special schools for primary-aged children and in residential schools for those with SLD. She also spent a year in a multi-disciplinary team to support the inclusion of children with learning difficulties in mainstream schools.

After spending three years as a Deputy Head in a large special school, she joined a local autistic society and for three years developed their training and educational information services, going on to become the first Principal of Coddington Court School for children aged 8–19 with ASD in Herefordshire.

She has also worked indirectly with adults and young people on the autistic spectrum.

Currently she works part-time as a Lecturer in ASD at Birmingham University with their web-based course (**www.webautism.bham.ac.uk**). She also works for Autism Cymru building up a series 3 National Fora for mainstream secondary school teachers, primary school teachers and special school teachers, to share good practice, and co-deliver LEA training with Maggie Bowen.

She has also worked in a consultancy role for Prior's Court School in Berkshire with teaching and care staff.

She tutors M.Ed dissertation students for the Course in ASD (Distance Learning) and is a member of the internationally respected Autism team, based at the University of Birmingham's School of Education, led by Professor Rita Jordan.

The Autism team has recently undertaken commissioned work to Develop an ASD information website and fact sheets for Primary Care Practitioners for NES–NHS in Scotland and a review of services for young people with Asperger syndrome in Northern Ireland, for the Northern Ireland Commissioner for Children and Young People (NICCY).

She is the book editor and an Editorial Board member of the *Good Autism Practice, Journal*. Lynn has built up a national profile of training in the importance of understanding the condition of autistic spectrum disorders for schools and care establishments.

Maggie Bowen

Maggie gained her academic and professional qualifications at universities in Aberystwyth, Leeds and Bangor. She began her teaching career in a school for children with severe learning difficulties (SLD), and went on to work as a Community Liaison Teacher for individuals with SLD. She has been a Team Inspector of secondary and special schools and a Threshold Assessor, and has worked as part of a multi-agency team and been responsible for developing a range of new services for individuals of all ages with a SLD.

She was Programme Leader for Special Educational Needs courses and the MA in Education at the North East Wales Institute of Higher Education (NEWI). In 2000, she worked as consultant/writer for the ACCAC (Wales) document '*A Structure for Success. Guidance on National Curriculum and Autistic Spectrum Disorders*'. She has worked for the Welsh Assembly Government (WAG) as Development officer for inclusion in Wales with a specific responsibility for Autistic Spectrum Disorders (ASDs), Able and Talented and SEN Training. She continues to work closely with the WAG on ASD matters.

She joined the team at Autism Cymru as Head of Public and Voluntary Sector Partnerships/Deputy CEO in January 2005. She has published on a range of SEN issues in books and journals, and is still committed to training and consultancy work with a range of practitioners from health, social services, education, the criminal justice system and the emergency services. She is a Registered Practitioner with the Higher Education Academy.

Hugh Morgan

Hugh Morgan has been Chief Executive of Autism Cymru, Wales's national charity for autism, since 2001. He had previously worked as the lead officer for the West Midlands Autistic Society (now autism.west midlands) for 14 years. Hugh started working in the learning disabilities and autism field as a nursing assistant in 1975 and has worked in a variety of hands-on settings with children and especially adults with autism. Hugh played a key role in the development of the autism training courses established by the University of Birmingham since 1990; and in 2003/4 was chair of the External Working Group for the autism strategy being developed by the National Assembly for Wales. Hugh is co-founder and co-editor of the *Good Autism Practice Journal* and an associate editor of *Autism* published by Sage/NAS. Hugh has professional and academic qualifications in psychology, social work, medical science and originally in nursing.

Acknowledgements

Our sincere thanks go to a range of people who have helped us gather evidence for this book, namely colleagues on the Webautism Team (**www.webautism.bham.ac.uk**), SNAP Cymru, Marilyn Sing at Cefnllys special nursery, Dr Elin Walker-Jones, Jude Bowen and NoMAD. We would also like to thank PAPA, Northern Ireland, for their inspiring approaches to individuals with ASD and their families.

How to use this book

This book is one in the series entitled 'The Autistic Spectrum Toolkit'. It focuses on the specific issues that can crop up in the early years of life, ranging from having suspicions about the young child displaying characteristics of ASD, through to common developmental differences displayed by the infant. Autism Cymru host a forum for teachers and workers in primary, and special schools, where they have the opportunity to share best practice and also their concerns about the young people in their care. The content of this book refers to some of the discussions that have taken place at these meetings and has therefore been shaped by the work of experienced practitioners.

The book is intended to cover many of the issues that have not been fully addressed in other works and we make brief reference to topics that are covered more fully elsewhere by giving the reader references to follow up by themselves.

Throughout the book, readers are asked to examine issues from the perspective of the individual with ASD, rather than adopt a traditional behavioural approach to the situation. Case studies of best practice and strategies suggested are designed to be of practical help to the reader. Readers are also given the opportunity to reflect on their practice and enhance their professional development by using the 'Reflective Oasis' contained in each chapter.

1

A guide to gaining a basic understanding of people on the autistic spectrum

> This chapter looks at the history behind the diagnosis of autistic spectrum disorders and some of the typical characteristics manifest in individuals with the diagnosis.

The condition of autistic spectrum disorders has had a relatively short diagnostic lifespan, compared with other disabilities (e.g. Down's syndrome, cerebral palsy) and it continues to have a range of different names (most with the term 'autism' mentioned somewhere). The main conditions of autism and Asperger syndrome were researched and outlined in the mid-1940s by two separate Austrian medical practitioners, Leo Kanner, a child psychiatrist, and Hans Asperger, a paediatrician. The condition of autism, or Kanner's autism as it is sometimes called, was published in English in 1943. The condition of Asperger (hard 'g') syndrome was published in German and reached English-speaking countries only in the 1980s when it was translated. A fuller historical picture can be gained from reading Wing (1996), Frith (1989) and Jordan (1999). It is possible that autism or its characteristics have existed through time (Frith, 1989; Waltz, 2005).

There is currently a range of professional views on giving a diagnosis of autism/Asperger syndrome/ASD. Look at what professionals and others have used to describe ASDs. These are all taken from literature and medical or educational notes.

What's in a name?

Kanner's autism
Classical autism
Childhood schizophrenia
Asperger syndrome
Autistic features
Childhood psychosis
Lack of theory of mind
Pathological demand avoidance
Idiot savant
Pervasive developmental disorder
Pervasive developmental disorder – NOS (not otherwise specified)
Central coherence difficulties
Semantic pragmatic disorder
Executive function deficit

The current terminology is 'autistic (or autism) spectrum disorder/s' (Wing, 1996).

Whatever the overarching label for the condition, there is a series of characteristics that are common to all – the triad of impairments (Wing, 1988) – three main areas of development where people with ASD manifest differences. These are:

- social interaction
- communication
- rigidity of behaviour and thought.

Social interaction

- Preference for individual activities
- Apparent aloofness
- Indifference towards others
- More adult-oriented than peer-oriented
- Likely to exhibit different spontaneous responses
- Passive acceptance of contact
- Lack of empathy
- Failure to appreciate significant others
- Poor understanding of social rules and conventions
- Inability to seek comfort at times of distress.

Wing and Gould (1979) believe that there is also a subgroup of three distinct character/behaviour types in social interaction.

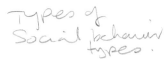

Types of Social behaviour types.

Aloof

Describes those people with ASD who behave as if you are not there, do not respond to your interactions and lead you to the place or activity that they want rather than requesting it.

Passive

Those who are completely passive in their interactions with others, will accept interaction and become a willing 'participant'.

Active but odd

Those who wish to have social contact but lack a means of initiating it in a socially appropriate way, so they may hold a gaze too long, sit too close or respond in an unpredictable way.

Communication

- Little desire to communicate socially
- Lack of understanding of non-verbal gestures of others
- Not appreciative of need to communicate information
- Idiosyncratic use of words and phrases
- Prescribed content of speech
- May talk at rather than to
- Poor grasp of abstract concepts and feelings
- Literal understanding of words and phrases
- Does not 'get' subtle jokes
- Will develop expression before understanding.

Rigidity of behaviour and thought

- May have stereotyped activities
- Can become attached to repetition of movement or certain objects or routines
- Complex order of activity
- Cannot deviate from one way of doing things
- May be tolerant of situations and then overreact to something minor

- May develop rituals that have to be completed
- Can have extreme physical rituals – e.g. spinning, rocking
- Can develop extreme behaviours to avoid certain stimuli.

These areas of difference in development have to be noted by the age of 3 years. Although there has been a greater willingness to diagnose young children in the last decade, many are not diagnosed until they are much older. A diagnostician will ask questions of parents/carers about their child's development before the age of 3. Professional reluctance to diagnose early may frustrate the needs of parents who are already suspicious about their child's development. However, the diagnosis is for a condition for which there is no known cure, so practitioners have to be absolutely sure that their assessment is accurate. Some of the characteristics of ASD could be the result of some other developmental delay. Chapter 2 deals with issues around diagnosis in more detail.

REFLECTIVE OASIS

Have you come across these characteristics in a child known to you?

How do these areas of impairment influence the way they relate to you?

Have you known a child who has not been diagnosed despite referral to a consultant?

What were their reasons for not diagnosing ASD?

Here are some common characteristics of people with ASD:

Social interaction

Limited tolerance of others
Inability to share or take turns
Inappropriate social behaviours

(Continued)

No desire to investigate or explore, unless it's an interest

Lack of empathy for others

Inability to know what others are thinking or feeling

Socially aloof or awkward

Restricted interests

Simple social actions are often a complicated process (organising themselves, personal space, dialogue)

May know some social conventions and apply them rigidly

Communication

Understands some basic instructions

Expresses own needs

Lack of desire to communicate

Lack of understanding of the attempts of others

No shared enjoyment of social situations

No use of gesture, intonation, non-verbal expression and inability to understand use of these by others

Cannot respond spontaneously

Appears not to 'hear' what has been said

Limited conversation repertoire

Talks incessantly on topic of interest and can manipulate conversations round to this topic

---

Rigidity of thought and behaviour

Finds it hard to separate fact from fiction

Difficulty in social situations that require a spontaneous response

Repetitive quality to interactions and routines

Will copy but not necessarily understand

Inability to see cause-and-effect of their own behaviour

Holds black-and-white views

Doesn't understand subtlety/sarcasm/jokes/irony

Cannot create spontaneously without a model or intensive input

May not transfer skills and concepts learned in one situation to other settings/people/topics

There is a general consensus of opinion that, in behavioural terms, there is no singular 'autistic' way of responding. These characteristics exist within all of us. The difference is that we 'neurotypicals' (NTs) are very good at disguising our stress, anxieties and weaknesses. Those on the autistic spectrum are not.

We have included the pertinent characteristics related to the defining characteristics of autistic spectrum disorders. We would refer readers to established references on the nature of ASD (Jordan, 1999; Wing, 1996; Cumine et al., 2000; Wall, 2004; Dickinson and Hannah, 1998) if they wish to gain a wider background to the condition and particular areas of the triad of impairments.

Points to remember

- The use of different terms for the same fundamental condition.
- The implications of the triad of impairments.
- Characteristics associated with ASD that can persist throughout life.

2

Identification and assessment

The identification and assessment of autistic spectrum disorders are covered fully in key texts on the condition (Wing, 1988; Wing and Gould 1979; Gillberg, 1991; Peeters and Gillberg, 1999). ASD is a pervasive developmental disorder, that is, a condition which becomes more apparent with the growth and maturity of the individual. It is not a condition that can be tested for during pregnancy or after birth because its precise cause is not yet known, although research continues to push back the boundaries of what we understand.

For some parents, the difference in the development of their young infant can be marked and worrying, particularly if they have had other children to make a comparison with. The key developmental differences become more apparent around the ages of 15–30 months of age where many milestones in development feature social and occupational skills. Many parents say that their child was a well-behaved baby who did not cry or want to be picked up all of the time. Others report a baby who never stopped crying.

Health visitors have a tool for screening youngsters with ASD, called the Checklist for Autism in Toddlers – CHAT (Baron-Cohen et al., 1992) and this will involve asking parents/carers some straightforward questions and observing the child in their home environment. There is a modified version of the CHAT – the M-CHAT (Robins et al., 2001) and a separate screening instrument for Asperger syndrome, called the Childhood Asperger Syndrome Test – CAST (Scott et al., 2002). Information gained from these screening

7

tools may be used to guide parents/carers toward requesting a referral from their GP to a team of professionals who can make an assessment. None of the current screening tools can currently claim 100 per cent accuracy, or 100 per cent sensitivity in picking up ASD conditions from a range of other childhood disorders.

Some of the typical differences in development that are noted around the toddler stage are:

- lack of recognition of significant others – mother, father, siblings, other children
- lack of wanting the attention of others in play, e.g. not holding up toys for approval or dropping toys for retrieval
- lack of joint attention – not pointing out; not making vocalisations for others to copy and make into a game
- lining/selecting or sorting to a predictable pattern
- slow development of a communication system – language is not developing or has developed in an unusual way – words are not used to convey meaning to others
- language development that has slowed or stopped
- indications of distress if routines are changed or situations or environments are new for them.

Current research suggests that ASDs have their roots in organic and genetic origins and they are not caused by poor parenting, social status, over-exposure to the TV or the MMR vaccine, to name but a few theories.

CASE STUDY

Why did our son, aged 14 months, not respond when we called his name, but he could hear a sweet wrapper from the next room?

Why, at the age of 20 months, did he speak in full sentences with perfect grammar in a BBC accent? (in the West of Scotland)

Why could he not tolerate a single word being changed when you re-read him a story?

Why did he never show any interest in the DIY his Dad was doing round the house or garden?

Why, at 24 months, could he name, at 200 yards, any make of car?

Why did he have difficulty playing with other children to the extent of biting them if they annoyed him?

(Continued)

Why did he have such a wonderful but quirky way of using or making up his own words for things?

Why, despite us suggesting he was socially not ready for school, were we told he was 'very bright but just a bit immature'?

Why did he feel the need to spend time hiding under his teacher's desk during the first few weeks in Primary One?

Why was his writing so bad but his reading so good?

Why did he have to have exactly the same packed lunch everyday for years?

Why would he never kick a ball or ride a bike, but would dress up as his favourite TV character and go on solitary 'quests'?

Why is he so phenomenally good at video games but has no sense of time passing?

Why did he not like opening his Christmas presents?

Why did he have to go through the whole of his primary schooling with various labels including 'spoilt', 'emotionally and behaviourally difficult' or 'having overprotective indulgent parents'?

Why did it take till he was aged 12 for us to be given the answer to all these questions that allowed us, and all those involved with him, to understand why and to move on?

Hindsight is a great thing!

(With grateful thanks to Alison and Jim Leask)

REFLECTIVE OASIS

Why might a parent miss some of the developmental differences in their young infant?

What possible explanations might a family and their relatives make for developmental differences?

How long would you wait before visiting your GP?

The diagnostic criteria

The recognised descriptors for diagnosis are contained in two separate medical reference books: the *ICD 10 – International Classification of Diseases Version 10* (1993), which is compiled by the World Health Organisation, and the *Diagnostic and Statistical Manual of Mental Health version IV* (1994), which is compiled by the American Psychiatric Association. The term 'autistic spectrum disorder', however, is not listed in either of these manuals, but the individual labels of autism, Asperger syndrome and pervasive developmental disorder not otherwise specified (PDD-NOS) are. Many diagnosticians will use these latter labels to define their conclusions as each represents further information on how ASD is manifest.

The issue of diagnostic labels and professional disagreement has an interesting history which has not been helpful to parents and those working with individuals with ASD. Further background on the history of ASD can be gained from Plimley and Bowen (2006b).

The diagnostic process

A diagnosis may be made by a paediatrician or child psychiatrist, and the child may be assessed by a multi-agency team including a health visitor, speech and language therapists, play therapists, occupational therapists, educational psychologists and others. The National Autism Plan for Children (NAP-C – NIASA, 2003) gives these guidelines:

- information on the individual must be gleaned from the major settings involved
- a history of development should be compiled
- observation of the individual needs to take place in settings that are familiar to them.

Additional information on the individual needs to be collated from key people/agencies on:

- levels of current functioning
- assessment of needs and strengths of the individual and their family
- assessment of sensory differences which can affect how the individual perceives and interacts with the world.

The above information forms a picture of the individual, with the views of their major carers. There is a number of diagnostic instruments to look at

ASD-specific factors in a developmental history and to guide assessment; please refer to the Glossary.

In recent years, more health trusts or authorities are able to offer a multi-disciplinary assessment and diagnostic service for ASD. This is a good way to form a holistic picture of the individual.

The benefits of a diagnosis include:

- mobilising services and agencies
- using appropriate interventions or strategies
- alerting key professionals to the needs of the individual and their family
- flagging up possible educational provision
- enabling the family to look for further information and to access support mechanisms.

The quality of services around the UK can be patchy, and parents, especially in rural areas, may have to travel long distances to see their diagnostician/s. The quality of follow-up from diagnosis can be equally patchy, with some medical professionals nominating educational placements for pre-school children at one extreme, to others delivering the diagnosis to anxious parents and then doing nothing else. The experiences of parents and carers at this very emotional and stressful time may colour their future views of professionals (Nally, 1999). Little wonder that parents/carers can seem anxious or needy, and desperate for information when they meet with subsequent professionals.

Statistics produced by the West Midlands Regional Partnership Project (2001) find some interesting time gaps between the age of the child at the time of parental suspicions of their child's development and having a diagnosis:

Age of child and parental/carer suspicions of their different development
N=443
59 had concerns from 0–12 months
178 from 12–24 months
123 from 24–36 months
83 from 36–48 months

Time gap between parent/carer's concerns and receiving a diagnosis:

N=451
78 had a gap of 12 months
133 of 12–24 months
90 of 24–36 months
59 of 36–48 months

51 of 48–60 months
40 waited between 10 and 16 years   *To long!*

Over half (63 per cent) of those interviewed in the Parent Carer Survey said that although they suspected that their child had ASD, nevertheless the professional diagnosis came as a crushing blow.

The survey also asked parent/carers what they needed most once they had had a diagnosis of ASD confirmed, and over half of them (56.9 per cent) requested more information in some form.

Post-diagnosis parent/carer needs were:

Information	32.9%
Advice/guidance	16.7%
Explanation	7.3%
Provision	5.6%
Prognosis	5%
Practical support for child and family	4.6%

The National Autism Plan for Children (NIASA, 2003) makes strong recommendations on improving the professional practice surrounding assessment and diagnosis and thereby improving the quality of the experience for the individual and parent/carer.

Post-diagnosis

Following diagnosis, parents/carers need to be linked up to the professionals who can offer further support. Some assessment and diagnostic centres will offer regular meetings to monitor the progress of the child. Some will give parents/carers information about local area support groups where they will meet other parents of children with ASD. Many parents/carers will need time to absorb and assimilate the information they have been given, and may want to return to their diagnostic team for further information, or they will go and trawl the Internet for as much information as they can get. For a more detailed focus on the experiences of parents of children with ASD, see Attfield and Morgan (2006).

Children diagnosed with ASD will need regular monitoring and follow-up of their development by professionals, including:

- health visitors
- Portage team

- pre-school multidisciplinary team
- child development centre
- psychology/speech therapy service
- health clinic
- GP clinic
- Social Services
- other paediatric services.

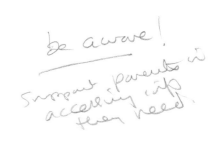

Be aware!

Support parents in accessing info they need.

Parents/carers can help enormously in this process by making observational records of their child to share with practitioners, that will note development in the areas of the triad of impairments. Parents may also want to examine more closely the impact of any sensory differences, and a useful profile is contained in the work of Bogdashina (2003, pp. 184–199.).

Observation of the child in different settings and with different people may also yield information not otherwise available to practitioners. Further approaches that give parents and practitioners a framework to monitor progress will be discussed in Chapter 6.

Points to remember

- The diagnosis of an individual with ASD needs to be a given after a multi-disciplinary assessment.
- The are strict criteria for diagnosis, either using the *DSM IV* or *ICD-10*.
- Further assessments can be carried out by other professionals.
- Sometimes parents can wait a long time to have their suspicions confirmed.

3

Family relationships

Parents do not plan to have a child with ASD. Rather all parents hope to have children who, as they grow older, will themselves become self-sufficient and independent, and have the desire to have their own children.

Parents experience a mix of emotions when they are told their child has a disability – especially when that disability is a 'hidden' one, like ASD. Parents find that they may have been lulled into a false sense of security regarding their child's development up to that point and now it's a 'double whammy' to find the perfect child they thought they had does not exist and they must adjust their aspirations and expectations accordingly. This is the start of a process which Attfield and Morgan (2006) describe as the 'parental emotional rollercoaster'.

For some parents who knew instinctively that 'something was not right', there may be relief at getting a diagnosis and being able to put a name to the difficulties they and the child are experiencing. They then discover they can do something about it by finding out about the condition and seeking information and interventions to help them deal with it. This becomes a coping strategy as much as the temporary withdrawal from the world other parents employ.

For parents, learning that their child has a disability – especially an autistic spectrum disorder – has, for many years, been viewed as equivalent to a bereavement. Practitioners need to be aware that parents of newly diagnosed young children with ASD need plenty of time and tolerance from others as they move from one stage to another. There is likely to be initial tremendous shock and denial.

'It can't be true! It's not fair … why him? … why us?' The sense of injustice and the anger, guilt and feelings of powerlessness and despair, may over-whelm parents before they finally come to accept their child for who s/he is. In time, without support and access to good information, the mental and physical health of parents may be affected, including:

- **Negative feelings** of helplessness, despair, being overwhelmed by cir-cumstances beyond own control
- **Stress** on parents, caused by the behavioural, social and communication problems of the child, and leading to a lack of confidence in their own ability to cope; and fear of the unknown, unexpected and unpredictable add to stress
- **Mental 'grind-down'** and stress of fighting for appropriate support and services for the whole family, and to obtain provision that meets the child's needs, advice on early intervention and an accurate diagnosis of the child's difficulties
- **Lack of sleep and opportunities to relax, leading to general physical exhaustion** because of child's needs and inadequate provision of respite care that would enable the carer to take a break from the 'juggling act' of chores and trying to lead a 'normal life'
- **Worries and anxieties** about the future, the child with ASD's progress, what's best for the child, the needs of other children in the family, possible marital breakdown and the deterioration of relationships between other family members.

[handwritten margin note: this can be mirrored in many diagnoses + even for parents where there is a much less severe learning difficulty]

How can practitioners working in the early years sector help?

[handwritten margin note: knowledgable, listening]

By spending time listening and empathising with the predicament and the stresses facing the family, and through a grounded understanding in ASD, you can explain and provide information to parents. Make sure that the most current information is available on local parent groups, sources of other local and national information which could be 'cherry picked' for the particular family to have facts and figures about ASD. Prepare a sheet about possible sources of information; refer to books such as *Living with Autism* (Attfield and Morgan, 2006) for helpful strategies which a parent might find of use. Make sure you stress some of the positive characteristics that a per-son with autistic spectrum disorder can bring to a family. By being calmly reassuring, you can play an important role in helping parents to understand that it is not their fault that their child has an autistic spectrum disorder and

[handwritten margin note: Simple info sheet pointing]

to help avoid the self-blame process that parents often go through. Even so, the reality is that, although it will be only parents and the wider family who themselves can come to terms with their situation and, indeed, at their own pace, you can help set the conditions for this process.

An important early message for parents of the newly-diagnosed child with ASD to realise is that they are not alone. They are, by absolute right, 'members' of a very large movement in the United Kingdom and wherever they should live in the UK, there are likely to be other families with a child with ASD not far away, and quite possibly there will be a local support group that they can join, and other parents whom they can talk to, who have been or are going through similar experiences.

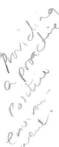

REFLECTIVE OASIS FOR PRACTITIONERS

How prepared are you to provide parents with concise, up-to-date and positive information to help signpost them through the minefield of newly-diagnosed ASD?

Younger siblings

There has been a spurt of interest in recent years in the siblings of children with ASD. There is a number of very good booklets aimed at younger siblings, such as Davis (1994b), the equivalent for the siblings of children with Asperger syndrome by the same author, and also the recent award-winning bilingual (Welsh/English) booklet *My Brother Gwern* (Walker-Jones, 2005), which are all well received by families, and in the case of the latter, can be obtained free of charge from Autism Cymru. Other useful books in this field are *My Brother is Different* (Gorrod, 1997) and *Everybody is Different* (Bleach, 2001).

In the younger age group, the focus of the literature has been to help the sibling to recognise and understand why their brother or sister is different. These booklets are about saying 'it is OK' and indeed to be proud of the brother or sister with ASD and of their idiosyncratic interests, at the same time acknowledging that it is also perfectly admissible to moan about the sibling with ASD and to find him/her 'a pain'. Conflict between siblings is natural, and siblings of children with ASD need not feel guilty for not always appreciating the foibles of their brother or sister.

For the older sibling, though, publications either on the web or indeed in book form are very hard to find. Yet as the child with ASD gets older, so do their siblings, and so the impact of ASD upon the sibling changes shape and has unforeseen implications.

Older siblings

The teenage brother or sister of the person with ASD may develop some pretty strong and often conflicting feelings and emotions and may become embarrassed and upset with the child who spoils games, destroys possessions, makes a noise and a mess, and causes disruption when out and about. Embarrassment may stem from what to tell their friends when they come home and they may choose not to bring friends home, with particular concerns at the time of the first girlfriend or boyfriend. Additionally, the brother or sister may feel s/he has to compete for parental attention and is 'second best' because so much time and energy have to be directed to the child with the disability and they may come to resent this. Parents need to be aware of placing a large burden of carrying parental hopes for the future upon the adolescent sibling as 'the successful one'. Paradoxically, it is the adolescent brother or sister who can become the fiercest defender of their sibling with ASD, and sometimes the reverse is also true, whereby the sibling with ASD idolises their non-ASD brother or sister.

How to help

- Siblings groups organised by a local autism society or other agency
- Being kept informed and involved in decisions about their sibling with ASD
- 'Special time' with parents away from the child with ASD
- Time and opportunity to have fun and live their own life, without guilt
- Acceptance that it is OK to express dissatisfaction with the sibling with ASD.

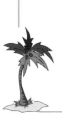

REFLECTIVE OASIS FOR PARENTS

How do you make sure that you give valued time and attention to your sons or daughters away from their sibling with ASD?

How do you acknowledge the role, feelings and worries of sons and/or daughters, and involve them in future planning and the present lives of their sibling with ASD?

Wider family issues

Some children are brought up by grandparents, other relatives or in extended families, while others are cared for by adoptive parents or foster-carers.

Grandparents can be especially important and may find it difficult to come to terms with the idea of ASD in the family, because they are worried not only about the welfare of their grandchild, but also the stress on their adult son or daughter of having a child with ASD. Yet, either or both grandparents can become extremely valuable support to the family with ASD. Grandparents may often take a very pragmatic approach to ASD in the family; after all, they have brought up their own children already and have a knowledge and a wise approach to life not always displayed by younger parents. Grandparents are good seekers and sifters of information on ASD which can be passed onto the parents, who should then expect to make their own decisions with total support from the grandparents. Grandparents can be great emotional props for their sons or daughters bringing up a child with autism, and can provide both moral and practical support and guidance in a crisis.

Points to remember

- Early years practitioners can play a key role in helping parents through the traumatic period following early diagnosis, with pre-planned information.
- Siblings of all ages need to understand how ASD affects their brother or sister and themselves, both now and in the future.
- All families are different and so the needs of individual families will differ.
- The wider members of the family can be of great support in terms of balance and objectiveness and during the occasional crisis.

4

Partnership with parents

Families do not ask for a lot from professionals. Indeed, their expectations tend to be realistic and reasonable. They do not ask for the earth and for all their problems to be solved by practitioners.

The core of the service that families look for during the early years may be summed up by the need to receive good information and guidance during and after assessment and diagnosis, to help them to have realistic expectations for the way forward; to know whom and what they are dealing with; to be listened to; and for their stories to be treated with respect and acknowledgement.

What Parents want.

This is not a one-way process, as practitioners within health, education and social services departments for their part have expectations as to how they should be treated by parents – not to be shouted at or threatened, to be acknowledged for their knowledge and experience; but also for it to be understood that they may have extreme demands upon their time.

The 'building blocks' of effective partnership

These principles are simple but can make all the difference. They include:

- mutual respect and tolerance
- a belief in the expertise, knowledge and experience of the other, leading to mutual understanding of where these overlap and complement each other

- a willingness and commitment to work together for the good of the child
- an honest and realistic approach
- positive communication
- co-operation towards shared goals
- flexibility
- listening skills
- encouraging strengths rather than always focusing on weaknesses
- accepting differences.

Attfield and Morgan (2006) say that:

> when there is a real sense of 'being in this together' the most successful partnerships are forged in the best interests of the child/adult with ASD at the centre of all the discussion. Let's not lose sight of the mental grind-down, over years, for the family of living with ASD and the battles it brings with it. Professionals who can stick with it for some of the ride with good humour and in the true spirit of partnership will be appreciated.

REFLECTIVE OASIS (FOR PRACTITIONERS)

Have you prepared helpful written information about ASD which families can take away with them?

How do you make parents aware that you acknowledge their experience and knowledge of their child?

Can you use and share your experiences of working with families with ASD to benefit other practitioners, including those from other disciplines?

REFLECTIVE OASIS (FOR PARENTS)

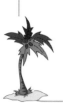

What do you know about the knowledge and experience of the practitioner?

Do you go into meetings with pre-conceived ideas about practitioners?

Parent partnership services

Local authorities today offer a free, confidential and impartial support service for families with children who have special educational needs (SEN) and of course, autistic spectrum disorders feature very prominently in this area. In terms of government policy, there is emphasis within the SEN Code of Practice for England and Wales upon the establishment of genuine partnership between practitioners and parents. However, the onus must be upon the 'professional' services to provide parents with as much prepared and evidenced-based information as possible to help them meet their individual needs.

The role of the voluntary sector and the importance of parents supporting parents

The voluntary (i.e. charity) sector is sometimes known as the 'Third Sector', as distinct from the public and private (profit-making) sectors. Many charities in all walks of life have been inspired and founded by people with the passion, commitment and motivation to ensure that vulnerable people are enabled to have a better quality of life in the future.

Autism charities (and there are many of them) are unquestionably among the most powerful of any of the Third Sector disability charities in the United Kingdom. Today, the family with a child with ASD is never going to be far from another family in a similar position, and there is a good likelihood that there will be a local autism charity with a parent support group, often led by parents themselves, wherever they live.

Indeed, the primary and most consistently long-lasting partnerships in ASD will lie between parents themselves, and not between them and practitioners. This will be a consequence of the lifelong commitment to ASD by the family, and the inevitable transience of practitioners who may, over time, get promotion or simply move on to other jobs and other roles.

So, the critical role played by the voluntary sector in providing an important and long-lasting service alongside the public sector has stemmed from parents themselves having been the prime movers and the most significant contributors. The voluntary sector can also play a very useful role in helping to bring about the development of services, and they add considerable weight and expertise to discussions with key representatives of the public services. Enormous strides have been made over the years by autism charities who have been the instigators of significant change; but equally we must not forget that there have been many in the public sector who have been both receptive and indeed very instrumental in bringing alongside the public services.

Points to remember

- Parents' expectations of practitioners tend to be both reasonable and realistic.
- Practitioners themselves look to be treated fairly by parents.
- Autism charities are often the source of the longest-lasting contacts, support and friendships for parents with children with ASD.

5

Multi-agency collaboration and service provision in the early years

This chapter examines ways in which professionals from health, education and social services can work together to provide a quality service for young children with ASD and their families. It gives a brief overview of the sorts of services that may be available and the advantages and disadvantages of each.

Multi-agency support

ASD can affect many aspects of the child's and family's life. It is possible that a family may have seen in excess of 20 professionals by the time their child is 5 (DfES, 2002a). General practitioners and health visitors might be the first to hear of parental concerns. This can lead to the involvement of professionals such as speech and language therapists (SALTs), clinical psychologists, occupational therapists and paediatricians.

Sometimes social services take the responsibility of assessing the family's needs and arranging short breaks or support workers/helpers for the child. Once the child is approaching school age, more education-related professionals will be introduced e.g. educational psychologists and advisory teachers. Throughout the process, the family may also be involved with voluntary organisations and support groups. With the potential involvement of so many people, clear communication between agencies is critical, to avoid repetition and confusion.

Effective collaboration

Each agency will have its own management structure, policy documents and funding arrangements. This can often make collaboration and the sharing of information difficult. Certain legislation, such as the Children Act (2004) assists by setting out the responsibility of councils to provide services to children in need and their families, to safeguard and promote their welfare. Local councils have a duty to work in partnership with families to provide those services to best meet needs. They also have a duty to set up and maintain a register of disabled children and publish information. The emphasis on Children's Services within the Act will impact on joint planning across agencies. A multi-agency web-based toolkit produced by DfES (2003) to assist in the process can be accessed from **www.everychildmatters.gov.uk/ multiagencyworking**

Local education authorities (LEAs) across England, Wales, Scotland and Ireland have been issued with a Code of Practice for children with additional needs which stresses the importance of multi-professional/multi-agency collaboration. The Education Act, Section 322 (1996), states that health authorities, subject to the reasonableness of the request and available resources, must comply with a request for help from an LEA, for children with special educational needs, unless they consider it is not necessary for the exercise of their functions.

Government initiatives such as Sure Start, Children's Fund, Neighbourhood Nurseries and Early Excellence Centres, work to support families and young children and emphasise the importance of the early years' development (NIASA, 2003). Lacey (2001) suggests that agencies are committed to working together and have strategies, such as bringing together joint committees, departments and teams with joint budgets.

Lacey (2001, p. 21) gives the following collaborative practice ideas:

- **Contracts and job descriptions** – to aid clarity and purpose in relationships between services.
- **Meetings** – giving teams the opportunity to talk and plan together and work alongside each other.
- **Structure** – facilitating meetings and joint working; encouraging the imaginative and flexible use of a professional's time. For example, using support workers to carry out daily speech and language therapy programmes under the weekly supervision and guidance of the SALT.

- **Key worker systems** – the appointment of a key worker or core team member who takes the responsibility for meeting the needs of individual children, using other members of the team in a consultative role.

Local area ASD co-ordinating group

Do we have one?

NIASA (2003) discovered that many local areas have some form of ASD planning or special interest group in response to the growing awareness of the needs of children with ASD and the level of demand for local services. They recommend the development of a multi-agency co-ordinating group to oversee setting up of local ASD services. The group will be made up of representatives from local parent and voluntary services that provide multi-agency assessments (MAAs), ASD interventions and support services.

Membership could include:

- representatives from local parent and voluntary services
- strategic managers from health, education and social services
- the named senior clinicians (or representatives) from health, 'local area based service': Primary Care Trust lead.

And the following professionals with ASD expertise:

- lead child health clinician and child development service manager of special needs register
- lead clinician – Child and Adolescent Mental Health Services (CAMHS)
- lead clinician – Community Learning Disability Services
- Speech and language therapists
- Occupational therapist
- Educational psychologist and/or LEA SEN officer
- Clinical psychologist
- Specialist teacher
- representative of therapeutic services (e.g. psychotherapy, music therapy)
- liaison health visitor
- ASD support worker and/or social services representative
- Administrative co-ordinator.

The **responsibilities** of the group should include:

- Liaison with and advice to local commissioning agencies.
- Local area training in ASD for all local community groups. The quality of the training should be monitored and/or externally validated and the training should meet agreed standards for different types and levels of training as set by national negotiation.
- Maintenance and supervision of the ASD database and special needs register.
- Auditing effectiveness of local identification, diagnosis and intervention services.
- Co-ordination of service planning and new developments informed by 'local' clinical need.
- Supporting provision of funding for, and access to, tertiary clinical services and establishing close links with specialist services to meet tertiary clinical needs.
- Co-ordination of academic and training links with a regional network to ensure that new developments inform local area practice. This is required at all levels from community-wide ASD awareness to specific diagnostic assessment practices employed and the portfolio of intervention expertise required within the local area.
- The development and planning of specific support/intervention within both specialist and mainstream settings on a local or regional basis.

CASE STUDY

Islington has a number of under-5s places for children with ASD that are defined as 'special' or 'additionally resourced' either in special schools or in an inclusive setting. The places are allocated in a co-ordinated multi-agency way. The Multi-agency Planning, Placement and Provision panel, an under-5's Advisory Group, brings together representatives from health, social services, education and providers. The group considers the needs of the children and information from parents/carers, and jointly decides how needs can be met. Each child's case comes to the group following a referral from the Child Development Team. They will have also been assessed by an educational psychologist. The group matches needs to provision and makes two or three recommendations to parents. The group will reconsider and attempt to offer alternatives if the family is not satisfied.

This service prevents a fragmented system and aims for rationality and the global view, taking into account all the professionals and agencies.

(From *ASD Good Practice Guide – Early Years Examples* **www.teach-ernet.gov.uk**)

REFLECTIVE OASIS

Consider a child you are working with.

How many other agencies or professionals are involved in meeting his/her needs?

What systems are in place to ensure that there is effective communication between all parties and that repetition and confusion are avoided?

Educational placement in the early years

The range of placements will vary across local authorities. Choosing the right educational placement can be difficult for parents, and service providers need to work together to help them make the right decision based on individual need – there is no 'one size fits all' solution. Parents might be influenced by the environment – is it a new build or does it look rather shabby? They might be concerned for the health and safety of their child. How many staff are available to help individual children? Professionals will need to be very sensitive to these concerns and appreciate that parents are only seeking what they consider to be right for their child.

Special schools specifically for children with ASD

Some LEAs have schools that cater for children with ASD, occasionally with residential provision. Private schools of this type also exist across the UK. The teaching staff will usually have a specialist knowledge and understanding of ASD. Their professional development is predominantly taken up with

ASD issues. Wall (2004) states that the school environment would revolve around daily routines, structure and visual clues. This offers reassurance and comfort to the children, enabling them to maximise their learning potential. Unfortunately, such schools may be situated far away from the child's home, separating them from their local community.

Special schools

Special schools cater for a wide range of additional learning needs. Classes are usually small and have a good pupil:staff ratio. Staff may not necessarily have had training in ASD. In this setting, children with ASD might find it difficult to cope in a class where there are high demands from other children. They may find noise levels distressing and may not have appropriate peer role models to encourage opportunities for social communication and interaction.

However, special schools vary in their policy and curriculum delivery and some may have special classes for children with ASD. In this instance, it is likely that staff would have had training in ASD-specific teaching strategies. Once again, such a placement may take a child away from the local community and parents might also feel isolated if they do not belong to a local family support group.

Resource bases attached to mainstream schools

Many LEAs have made provision for children with ASD in the mainstream primary school. This may still mean being educated outside their local area. The resource bases will usually have appropriately qualified staff, and the structures, routines, curriculum and environment to maximise learning potential. Opportunities for children to participate in the life of the school would be carefully planned, and based on individual need and tolerance levels. Ideally, all staff outside the base will have a knowledge and understanding of ASD.

Mainstream schools and early years settings

Many children with ASD have their needs appropriately met in their local mainstream provision. For early years, this would usually be in the nursery class on either a full- or part-time basis and then later in Reception class. In some instances, children may have access to a full- part-time support worker or teaching assistant. Wall (2004) points out for more able children with ASD, such a placement can be highly successful provided that staff are suitably trained and are flexible in their approaches. The placement would also have benefits for other children in the class, giving them a clearer understanding of individual differences.

Assessment centres

Such centres are designed to be short-term placements where children undergo a detailed assessment, in order to inform long-term planning. Any movement from this sort of placement to another following assessment would need to be considered well in advance. Assessment centres are not ASD-specific and so the issues would be the same as for the special school.

Home-based programmes/applied behavioural analysis centres

Some parents fight for their child to be educated using a particular approach or intervention. These approaches are discussed in Chapter 10.

Thoughts for early years providers

In terms of early years provision, it is crucial that service providers consider:

- all children with ASD are unique and so any placement or intervention should be based on individual need
- staff involved should be adequately trained
- specialist input may be needed from a range of providers
- parents should be fully informed about their child's provision via regular meetings, telephone calls and home–school diaries
- information leaflets and letters provided for parents should be written in clear, jargon-free language(s)
- the child's learning targets should be reviewed regularly
- where a number of practitioners is involved in the learning process, there should be clear lines of communication and consultation
- any transition from one service to another should be carefully planned.

CASE STUDY

Working together in mainstream schools to meet the needs of children with ASD

Some mainstream schools in Rhondda Cynon Taff have taken part in Autism Cymru's Inclusive Schools and ASD Research and Training Programme. As part of the Programme, all staff undergo awareness training of ASD and carry out an audit of their school environment to ascertain whether or not it is 'ASD friendly'. As a result of the audit, schools recognised the importance of making special arrangements at break times and lunch times for pupils with ASD, and the need to think creatively about making a 'safe haven' for pupils to reduce stress levels. Examples included the use of a library area with cushions and blinds for relaxation, and a screened-off part of the classroom with a bank of relaxing resources to accommodate individual sensory preferences.

REFLECTIVE OASIS

Make a list of the strengths of your early years setting for a young child with ASD.
Then consider the shortfalls in your setting.
What can you do to improve things?

Points to remember

- Multi-agency collaboration is crucial in the delivery of high-quality services.
- Professionals should work closely with parents and be sensitive to their requests.
- A number of educational placements can exist for young children with ASD – there is no 'one size fits all'.
- Staff working with children with ASD should be suitably trained in order to meet their needs.

6

Using a statutory framework to enhance service provision in the early years

This chapter examines the SEN Code of Practice (DfES, (2002b)/WAG, 2002) and its impact on service provision for young children with an ASD. It gives an overview of the graduated response, statutory assessment and the role of the special needs co-ordinator (SENCo) in the early years. It suggests how practitioners could write Individual Education Plans. Finally, it discusses the implications of the 2001 Special Educational Needs and Disability Act (DfES, 2001).

The SEN Code of Practice

In 2002, the Welsh Assembly Government and the Department for Education and Skills introduced a revised version of the Special Educational Needs Code of Practice (1994). The revised Code places a greater emphasis on parental involvement and pupil participation, and introduces a different approach to assessment of need (the graduated response). It offers practical advice to local education authorities (LEAs), maintained schools, early years settings and others, on carrying out their statutory duties to identify, assess and make provision for children's special educational needs.

The graduated response in the early years

The graduated response to service provision recognises the varying levels of need and support among children. No two individuals with ASD are the same; each will respond in their own unique way to different teaching approaches and levels of support. The graduated response comprises:

- Early Years Action
- Early Years Action Plus
- requests for statutory assessment
- statements of special educational needs

The graduated response can be viewed as an approach to a continuum of need, and the more flexible and responsive early years' practitioners can be, the more likely it is children with ASD will make progress. Strands of action are introduced so that more suitable interventions can be used to meet increasing need.

If a young child with ASD is not making progress, despite receiving some differentiated learning opportunities, intervention through Early Years Action may be necessary. Often this is will be the case for a youngster with a diagnosis of ASD or one who is currently undergoing assessment. It is important to note that individual need rather than a definitive label should be the main consideration. Some young children without a recognised label of ASD may respond well to the strategies used with pupils with ASD.

Intervention will be required if the child is making little or no progress in learning skills, and if behaviour management techniques are having no effect. Sometimes in the early years, young children with ASD are described as naughty and aggressive, when inappropriate behaviour may be the only means of indicating how distressed they are feeling.

At Early Years Action, the SENCo will need to work closely with early years' practitioners, parents and the child to develop an individual plan. It may be necessary to seek information from relevant professionals in health and social services or engage the services of specialist as a consultant to prevent the future development of more significant needs.

If a child does not make progress, seeking help and advice from specialist support services for ASD may be needed in a more intensive way. Such 'specialists' may be able in a more intensive way to advise on new ideas for individual education programmes (IEPs), specialist resources and teaching strategies. The advice and support that can be offered will vary according to local policy and procedure. If a child requires support at this level, s/he will be referred to Early Years Action Plus of the graduated response.

During this stage, parents, carers and the child (where appropriate) should be consulted. Additional advice or support should not be sought without parental consent.

In Northern Ireland, a five-stage approach to assessment is used (DENI, 2005 a, b). This follows a similar format to the graduated response in terms of service provision.

REFLECTIVE OASIS

In meeting the needs of young children with ASD, what targets do you set in relation to:

- assessment, planning and review?
- additional human resources?
- curriculum and teaching methods?
- grouping for teaching purposes?

Statutory assessment and statements of special educational needs

Some pupils with ASD will not make adequate progress at Early Years Action Plus, and parents and practitioners may decide to make a referral for statutory assessment. The early years setting may have to provide evidence that attempts made to improve progress have failed. However, parents of children with ASD may feel dissatisfied with the provision in early years and make a direct referral for statutory assessment and subsequently a statement of special educational needs for their child. Parents are at liberty to take a local education authority to the Special Educational Needs Tribunal if the LEA refuses this request.

A statement is a legal document that describes a child's special educational need and the range of available provision to meet those needs. Written advice is gathered from parents, professionals in health, social services and education. For some parents, a statement is a legal safeguard and a security that their child's needs will be met and reviewed on a regular basis.

However, there is currently a great debate around statutory assessment and statements of SEN, e.g. Audit Commission (2002); Estyn (2004); Welsh Assembly Government (2006a) whether statements exist or not. It will be the responsibility of early years practitioners to see that any assessment process adopted is responsive to, and supportive of, the needs of children and their families and provides the assurance that needs will be met, monitored and reviewed, and lastly, that there is a genuine teamwork and partnership between all involved.

In Scotland, a staged intervention system has been adapted with Co-ordinated Support Plans for children with complex educational needs which require continuing review (Scottish CCC, 1999).

CASE STUDY

One LEA has reduced the numbers of statements it issues without complaints from parents. It has been successful because they have made sure that parents are very well informed about the process and the fact that both school and LEA are able to meet needs at Early Years/School Action Plus. The progress of each child is monitored on a termly basis and parents are invited to attend the review. This gives parents the opportunity to raise any concerns on a regular basis.

REFLECTIVE OASIS

What systems does your setting have in place to reassure parents that their child's needs are being met, monitored and reviewed, regardless of whether the child has a statement of special educational needs?

Writing Individual Education Plans (IEPs)

It is very likely that practitioners will need to consider writing an IEP for young children with ASD and it is important that this is done with reference to the triad of impairment. Targets will therefore focus on communication, social interaction, imagination and flexibility of thought.

The ASD Toolkit (PAPA, 2003) produced in Northern Ireland provides excellent guidance on writing IEPs. Practitioners complete an observation profile to provide a baseline against which progress can be monitored and reviewed (see Table 1). The profile can be used to identify targets and consider appropriate strategies for intervention. Although young children may have the same core difficulties, each will be unique in his/her own characteristics.

The profile should contain the following information:

- contact information – name, setting details
- assessment details such as reports from a range of professionals outlining issues around the triad
- the learning profile of the child, to highlight any uneven patterns in skill acquisition
- strengths and interests
- needs based on the above.

It will be necessary to prioritise needs – all difficulties cannot be solved at once. The toolkit suggests that practitioners should follow this procedure:

- **List assets** – what are the positives about the child? Maybe s/he works well in a small group or responds to a one-to-one working relationship.
- **List barriers to learning/socialising** – What is the child not so good at? Maybe s/he loses attention if s/he is not in a one-to-one working situation.
- **Agree priority problem** – What do you consider to be the biggest problem? Perhaps the child is unaware of road danger.
- **State the desired target/objective/outcome** – What do you want the child to do instead? For example, do you need to make him/her more aware of common dangers?
- **IEP signposts to planning** – How can you help the child achieve her/his new targets? For example, you may need to use social stories (Gray, 1994; **www.graycenter.com**) to teach her/him about dangers.

The person responsible for monitoring and reviewing the IEP will vary and will be influenced by the child's needs in relation to the graduated response. Often the early years' special needs co-ordinator and the practitioner directly involved with the child will work together and alongside parents/carers.

Targets/objectives should be phrased in a way that is positive, emphasising the acquisition of new skills. The Toolkit offers the following example:

John will have less than two tantrums each week for four consecutive weeks. [negative]

becomes

John will go to a specified area during most of his tantrums for four consecutive weeks. [positive]

Table 1: The IEP process flowchart (ASD Toolkit, 2003)

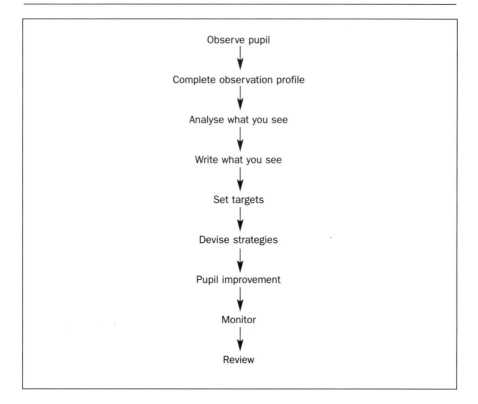

ACCAC(2002) recommends the use of SMART targets – specific, measurable, achievable, realistic and timed.

> **CASE STUDY**
>
> ***CASE STUDY: EXAMPLE OF AN IEP (with thanks to Autism Northern Ireland (PAPA))***
>
> ***Individual Education Plan***
> ***Personal Information***
>
> ***Name   DOB***
>
> ***Date:***
> ***Objectives of Provision***
>
> *To help XXXX to develop social and communication skills to interact with her peers and adults*

Targets
- *Sit alongside other children during break/lunch times*
- *Take turns with adult to build a Lego tower (Duplo) of 20 bricks*

Strategies and Resources
- *Small groupings at individual tables for break times and lunch. Seating arrangements for children same each time (visual cues), Teacher to make/written comments diary of progress*
- *Turn-taking activities for giving out food and drink*
- *Use of PECs or other picture symbols to communicate preference*
- *Designated time for 1:1 with two different adults to build Lego tower. Use of a recording chart*

Staff Involvement
Mrs X (Nursery Teacher)
Miss Y (Support Worker)

Specialist Involvement (if appropriate)
Advice from Speech and Language Therapist re PECs

Parental Involvement
Parents are to be kept informed of progress. Mother to encourage turn-taking activities at home and use Picture Symbols for communication. Similar procedures will be followed during family meal times.

Pastoral/Medical Requirements
XXX is sensitive to touch. Adults will need to be aware of this when prompting during brick building exercise.

Monitoring/Review Arrangements
XXX will be recorded on a daily basis and progress reviewed every two weeks.

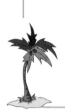

REFLECTIVE OASIS

How do you organise your IEPs?

Are the headings similar to those above?

Do you take into account targets directly related to the triad of impairments?

How do you monitor, review and adapt your IEPs?

The role of the special educational needs co-ordinator (SENCo) in the early years

It is the responsibility of the SENCo to liaise with parents and other professionals. The SENCo should advise and support other members of staff in the setting and ensure that appropriate IEPs are in place. It is their duty take the lead in the assessment of a child's strengths, areas for development and to plan future support with colleagues. SENCos should keep a record of children at Early Years Action and Early Years Action Plus.

CASE STUDY

The SENCo in one infants school has developed a resource bank for colleagues, consisting of documentation for assessment, best practice guidance, worksheets, and details of different disorders including ASD, with a list of appropriate contacts. Within the resource base there are custom-made pro formas for IEPs, reviews and contact with parents. The bank also houses a battery of assessment tests that the SENCo undertakes with pupils.

(With thanks to Hafod y Wern Infants, Wrexham)

REFLECTIVE OASIS

How does the SENCo in your setting support colleages in planning Individual Education Programmes for youngsters with an ASD?

The Special Educational Needs and Disability Act (DfES, 2001)

SENDA (DfES, 2001), which amended the Disability Discrimination Act (Department of Work and Pensions,1995), makes it unlawful to discriminate against children or young people with a disability and prospective pupils in relation to admissions, the provision of education and exclusions. It also requires the responsible body for a school to take steps to ensure that pupils with a disability are not substantially disadvantaged, and are included in all aspects of school life, unless there is evidence that this would not be in the child's best interest. If a child with ASD is excluded from any activity, the staff must ensure that a risk assessment has been undertaken to justify this action.

CASE STUDY

Joe attends a resource base for young children with ASD within a primary school. He is a Year 2 pupil. The school had arranged an outing for other Year 2 pupils in the school to visit to the zoo. Joe's mother was upset to discover that her son would not be going on the trip with his peer group. The school informed her that they had carried out a risk assessment for Joe to go on the trip and that he would need one-to-one supervision. Joe's mother said she would happily provide the supervision. All those involved considered this to be a reasonable adjustment and Joe went on to have a very happy time at the zoo.

REFLECTIVE OASIS

What systems are in place in your setting to ensure that youngsters with ASD have equality of opportunity?

Points to remember

- Early years providers must pay due regard to the guidance set out by their respective countries.
- The graduated response is an approach used in England and Wales to meet a continuum of need.
- Parents/carers need information, support, guidance and reassurance during the assessment process and should be consulted on any action that may take place.
- Individual Education Plans (IEPs) should take into consideration the triad of impairments.
- Every early years setting should have a designated person (SENCo) with a responsibility for pupils with additional needs, including ASD.
- ASD is a disability and so staff must give consideration to SENDA in terms of fair access and inclusion.

7

Social skills training – self-help skills

The key defining features of the triad of impairments (Wing, 1988) will have a marked impact in all areas of social skills at all stages in life. This chapter examines some of the features that can act as an alert to parents/carers that their child may be following a different developmental path from what is typical, and offers strategies that can help social skills development.

Early infanthood

ASD is a pervasive developmental disorder, rather than a congenital condition (that someone is born with). Therefore, it is highly unlikely that a newborn baby will manifest the differences associated with the triad. Many parents say that they first began to suspect that their child was developing differently when they were between 12 and 18 months. This also coincides with the rapid development of language and play skills.

Differentiation of behavioural development

There are some behaviours which can alert the parent to developmental differences:

- Lack of interest in others
- Not 'hearing' what others are saying – paying little attention to the communication of others.

Most very young children will cue into the sound of a human voice and as they grow, will turn in the direction of that voice. Often they can pick out a voice or a human shape above other distractions and seem to know instinctively to give their attention to humans.

The child with ASD may be more preoccupied in a toy or patterns or something they have picked up, and appear not to notice or hear humans. Many parents have their child's hearing tested as a first medical procedure.

- Lack of recognition of significant others – mother, father, siblings, other children
- Indications of distress if routines are changed or situations or environments are new for them.

The young baby will be able to recognise the shape and smell of familiar people, before their sight is acute enough to see particular features. This skill develops first with their primary care giver (PCG) – usually the mother, but not always; and the baby will make the connection between the human and the likely activity – feeding, washing, changing, etc. As their sight develops, the baby will recognise significant people in their lives and demonstrate their security by allowing cuddles and close contact. This recognition assists them in picking out a familiar voice, constraining their spontaneous activity and encouraging them to communicate and entertain, or make their needs known. Most young children can be taught to know the difference between safe and dangerous, and between a stranger and someone you know. Very young children also gravitate to other youngsters as potential playmates.

The young child with ASD may regard all people as strangers who pose a potential threat to their comfort and security. Regular routines, such as those mentioned above, will provoke a response as if this is a new (and threatening) activity and they will become distressed and/or resistant. For the PCG, this can be worrying and upsetting as the chain of events from the baby being distressed and resistant will provoke the PCG into finding ways to pacify and comfort. This might lead to more distress and resistance. In extreme circumstances, the child with ASD may dictate a family life where everyone is afraid of provoking a distressed reaction. If the youngster does not respond to attempts to play or communicate, then the richness of early language experiences (lap-play, exaggerated reactions, anticipation and peek-a-boo games) will also be lost.

- Lack of wanting the attention of others in play, e.g. not holding up toys for approval or dropping toys for retrieval by others.

Before the age of 12 months, babies will vocalise or make actions that 'grab' our attention. Much of this is aimed at their PCG but when one observes young children in shops and restaurants, they appear to have this homing device for anyone who will give them eye contact. We, for our part, automatically respond with a funny face, a gesture or vocal encouragement. And so the dance continues.

The child with ASD can begin to develop these skills and then suddenly lose them. Parents often report that they fail to develop that homing instinct in the first place. They can appear to exist in a vacuum with their own interests and activities that rarely includes other people. They can become very distressed by changes in routines or environments, or when things that they anticipated do not happen.

- Lack of joint attention – not pointing out; not making vocalisations for others to copy and make into a game.

Following on from the point above, most typically developing youngsters will develop particular vocalisations when they want to share your attention. PCGs will know what different tones and noises mean for their child. They seem instinctively to develop a pointing or similar gesture that can be used to draw attention to something outside of their physical range too, and may use pointing and a noise to further underline their interest. PCGs will have routines, rituals, songs and rhymes that they use to encourage their child to vocalise and mimic actions. Many early play experiences for the child will involve games that the child can anticipate the actions for – hiding, covering up, picking up on exaggerated actions.

The child with ASD may not want or like this type of attention and because of their lack of interest in people, may not engage in any of the above activities.

- Playing with mechanical objects in a rote fashion (not varying play activity)
- Lining up or selecting or sorting to a predictable pattern
- Preoccupation with particular toys or activities that involve repetitive body movements.

Young children develop their play interest by engaging in play as a social activity. Toys for very young children invite their attention and will often have activating mechanisms that require someone 'in the know' to wind up, shake, pull or push the toy to make it move. Pretend and symbolic play is also a shared activity, or else the child may not know how to use one object to represent another or to spontaneously use a particular costume to make them into another person. Most typically developing children love the surprise element of having a new toy or receiving gifts on their birthdays – this involves social contact and social pleasure.

The child with ASD likes the familiar and they also like things that they can manipulate for themselves, by themselves. They can become preoccupied with very detailed mechanical toys and seek to replicate that experience when they find other toys. Often this can be rotating car wheels or engaging in play that requires their movement in a repetitive way – like spinning or hand flapping or clapping. When observing the play of a child with ASD, there does appear to be an unvaried quality to it. This may persist through life. Or they will enjoy a particular song or video over and over again. De Clercq (2001) says that her son equated turning round and round to the concept of being married – because in the Disney's *Cinderella* that's what she and Prince Charming did when they danced at their wedding. These misconceptions can build up from a lack of social understanding. For the child who likes particular patterns and arrays of objects, these become touchstones of security for them, and to alter or move their arrangement can mean major distress.

- Slow development of a communication system; language is not developing or has developed in an unusual way; words are not used to convey meaning to others
- Language development that has slowed or stopped.

The typically developing child will have their own means of communication before their first birthday using vocalisation, intonation, different sounds for different meanings. Vocalisation develops into near-word utterances which then form the basis of an early single-word vocabulary and then phrases. Thereafter, use of communication builds alongside their rapid comprehension of what is said to them. In typically developing children, the development of understanding the spoken word precedes their use of first words, and very young children will look at an object that is being talked about quite a while before they articulate its name.

The child with ASD can develop the use of language before comprehension and can articulate some sophisticated language which does not tally with their understanding. ASD is the only condition where language can develop before comprehension (Jordan, 1999). Echolalia is the repetition of words, sayings or phrases without an understanding. Echolalia can be a feature of ASD. Many people with ASD will say words or phrases over to themselves for the sheer pleasure of the sound, or to de-stress themselves. They will repeat a phrase that is associated with an particular emotion or action – 'Don't do that!' when they are about to engage in something that they should not. PCGs report that their child can sound like a 'little Professor' because their language sounds so sophisticated, but often the understanding is missing. Some people with ASD do not develop a spoken language at all, but can use gesture and demonstration to get their point across. Others work particularly well with a symbol or photograph as a means of communication. Filipek et al. (1999) say that the following communication 'red flags' are cause for referral in early childhood:

At 12 months – no babbling, no pointing or other use of gesture
At 16 months – absence of single words
At 24 months – absence of two-word phrases
Any loss of language or social skills at any age.

REFLECTIVE OASIS

Think about a child that is known to you. If you have known this child since they were under 2, consider the communication 'red flags' that Filipek et al. (1999) have outlined.
Analyse the child's communication development and try to pinpoint when they started to babble, use single words and two-word phrases.

Pre-school

Early years provisions are intended to build upon the skills and interests of the child, to begin more formal learning experiences and to build up concentration and attention spans. They also focus on socialisation with others of their age. For many children with ASD, the pre-school setting can represent a confusing world. They may respond with anxiety and fear which is then manifest by becoming more involved in self-stimulatory behaviours, e.g. spinning, rocking or making repetitive noises. Such behaviours may be a means of calming down.

By the age of pre-school or nursery placement, most children will have mastered the self-help skills of eating, sleeping through the night and be toilet trained by day. Acquisition of these skills can become developmental sticking points for the pre-school child with ASD.

Food

For children who are 'stuck' on a particular food, texture or method of presentation, the following guidelines may help.

Use visual prompts (photos, objects of reference) to prepare the child for eating.

Be aware of smells and textures – present different foods but with same texture.

Don't enforce eating together; focus on them sitting at the table with their meal as the first goal.

Try to ensure their diet is balanced, and take nutritional advice from the doctor or pharmacist.

Lay their place at the table in the same way every time.

Have the same range of condiments.

Make basic rules and keep to them – like 'sit and eat/drink': do not allow eating or drinking under any other circumstances.

Look to extend tolerance of tastes/textures gradually.

Develop a social story (Gray, 2000) around food routines.

There are some individuals with ASD who will eat a restricted diet because of particular allergies or toxins (Williams, 1996). Typical foods that are avoided are wheat or dairy products (Le Breton, 2001; Jackson, 2002). Parents of children with ASD may want to try gluten-free foods (to avoid wheat) or casein-free foods (to avoid dairy), and the availability of 'free-from' products at the supermarket can make this easy. Any care or educational setting for the young child with ASD will need to work alongside parents if an exclusion diet is being tried.

Some parents will opt to try an additive-free diet such as omitting salicylates or yeast or artificial colourings, or using mineral and vitamin supplements such as Vitamin B or omega 3 and 6 fish oils. The Autism Research Centre at Sunderland University (**http://osiris.sunderland.ac.uk/autism/**) has built up a range of data to support the view that some exclusion diets do work with some kinds of gut disorders in individuals with ASD. Parents who are studying on the Webautism course at the University of Birmingham (**www.webautism.bham.ac.uk**) have reported varying degrees of success with different food regimes and recommend professional advice.

Toilet

For children who are not making the connection between the sensations of urinating or defecating and using a potty, the following guidelines may help.

Make using the potty into a routine.

Always use the same toilet or potty in the same place.

Develop a script and make it into a story.

Use photos, pictures or objects to back up the information.

Give little or no reaction to 'accidents'.

Use strong rewards – a twiddle of a string or five minutes' trampolining, instead of 'well done' or a hug.

Children with ASD can develop some fastidious toilet habits. Be aware of any subtle changes in the routine, because they can upset a skill that is being acquired. Changing the toilet request or sensory overloads, e.g. sudden noises, may cause distress and a fear of using the toilet or potty. Children may sometimes defecate only in a nappy and can 'save up' the contents of their bowels for a long time until a nappy is put on. Routines and rewards, as well as maintaining a strict continuity in request and circumstance, may help get around these inflexibilities.

CASE STUDY

Hon Li is a 3-year-old boy who is doubly incontinent and depends on his Mum to anticipate and respond to all of his primary care needs. Hon Li enjoys collecting shells and gets very engrossed in his collection. Sometimes he will carry on playing until it is too late and he has soiled himself.

The pre-school setting worked with Mum to chart when and how often Hon Li urinates and defecates. They devised a chart using Hon Li's love of shells to show him when he would be put on the potty and for how long. They used a simple egg timer to mark the passage of time. While he was on his potty, a story about shells was read to him and the reward for using the potty was immediate time to play with his shell collection. Hon Li became continent of urine within a week.

Sleep

For children who are unable to go to sleep, or to sleep through the night, the following guidelines may help.

Clear structure and routine and time for going to bed.

Bed is for sleeping in.

But bedroom can have other activities in for independent occupation.

Check preferences and sensory overload or sensitivity – take out over-stimulating materials and consider the decor.

Consider relaxation exercises.

Develop a time-related, rules-bound approach.

Be clear in your own mind and stay consistent.

Points to remember

- Each child with ASD is an individual with their own particular tastes, habits and routines.
- Careful observation of the child during routines may yield information on their likes and dislikes.
- It may also give information on hitherto unknown sensory differences.
- Approach learning of new self-help skills with an open mind and a willingness to help the child achieve as much independence as possible.

8

Managing behaviour

It is a fallacy that everyone with an ASD will have some form of difficult or challenging behaviour. What one will see in people with an ASD are some behavioural extremes which are not tempered by social understanding, emotion or social rules. This is what is missing at the core of the disorder – the social factor that can prohibit or at least inhibit behaviours.

There are no 'typical' behaviours in ASD, although people mistakenly believe that rocking, spinning and pacing up and down, as well as the more challenging biting, spitting and lashing out exist as a feature of ASD. These behaviours may signal sensory overload or a situation of unbearable stress. The behavioural manifestation is an attempt to control the situation and/or de-stress. For the majority of these behaviours, there is an attempt to communicate something. For us – neurotypicals or NTs – we can exhibit these behavioural extremes at times of stress or anxiety – exactly as for those with ASD.

Consider:

- An overwhelming sadness you have felt – crying, rocking, stroking may have helped you.
- A time of extreme stress – pacing, checking/re-checking or inability to respond to others may have been your response.
- A time when you felt physically threatened – did you also respond physically?

- A time when you were repeatedly misunderstood – shouting, non-verbal aggression, physical approaches may have been a more effective form of communication.

Cumine et al. (1998) say we often look at the behaviours of the person with Asperger syndrome, instead of how the person may be thinking and reasoning. They recommend applying an 'Asperger lens' to situations when we analyse them. So we will look at common early years behaviours and apply an ASD lens.

An insistence on sameness and familiarity

ASD lens

The individual will take comfort and security in a world they struggle to understand by recognising familiar patterns and routines. Changing the route to the supermarket or wearing a new pair of shoes may mean that they will feel insecure and stressed. Gradual introduction to a change or having a system which signals change in advance (TEACCH; see Chapter 9) may make adjustment easier.

A need to be shown how to do something they had previously been able to do independently

ASD lens

PCGs report that the child can 'forget' or 'lose' skills they had previously acquired. Often this can happen when the child is feeling under stress (don't we get confused when things change?) or the loss may be longer term. The individual with ASD may have to overlearn new skills and knowledge, and try the same things out in a variety of different settings with different people because they have not generalised the skill.

Crying or screaming for no apparent reason and for long periods of time

ASD lens

This is often their only way to communicate when everything is going wrong, or is getting too much for them. PCGs and practitioners may find that once the child has a more efficient means of communicating – using words, pointing or a scheme such as the Picture Exchange Communication System (Bondy and Frost, 1994) – these episodes diminish.

Refusal to be comforted

ASD lens

We instinctively believe that close physical contact will calm. For a person with ASD, physical proximity of others may be a difficulty; unanticipated physical contact can be alarming; the feel of another body, acting as an unintentional restraint, may be frightening.

Using a physical means of getting your attention

ASD lens

It is quite common for individuals with ASD to use people as a conduit to what they want – e.g. leading you to the desired toy that is on the top shelf. Lots of typically developing youngsters will do this too. It is also a stage of typical development to throw a tantrum until someone does something ('terrible 2s'). This may persist into adulthood for some people with ASD. If a scream or a bite gets the required result, that is what they will use. Taking someone to something that you want, is an indication that the stages of a communication system are understood – there has to be an object, another person and a desire to communicate, but the child is lacking the use of language or a recognisable system. Pointing is something that may have to be taught, but can be used very effectively.

It may be necessary to combine strategies in order to counteract deeply entrenched and potentially dangerous behaviours (Dickinson and Hannah, 1998). Try to look objectively at what the causes of the challenging behaviour are. Dickinson and Hannah (1998) say that compiling a diary over a prescribed period may help you to pinpoint some things that have changed for the child. The environment itself can often trigger poor behaviours that NTs are unaware of. Sudden noise, changes of décor, new smells and new furniture often trigger behaviours that are a response to new sensations. A minimal-stress environment may have to take those factors into account. You should also look at ways of communicating familiar routines and events, as well as changes to the child.

Using an ASD lens may help us to reframe the way in which we view behaviours that have appeared to be challenging.

> **CASE STUDY**
>
> Charlie always enjoyed his visits to see his grandma. He loved travelling on the bus with his Mum. He looked out for familiar sights on the way and always commented on post boxes, police cars and traffic lights. He always said familiar sayings to himself ('green lights', 'post a letter'), and his Mum's attention was not needed. One day on a visit Charlie threw himself on the pavement by Grannie's, kicking and screaming, saying over and over 'No Grannie, no Grannie'. His Mum could not get close to him and as people went past, they stared and tutted. Charlie would not get up for his Mum. Fortunately his Grannie came out to help, and Charlie started to calm when he saw her. When he was up on his feet, he still would not follow Mum and Grannie into her house. His anxiety started to rise again and he began to cry. Mum and Grannie could not work out what had upset him. They brought a drink and snack out into the front garden because Charlie was so reluctant to go inside. Grannie started to talk about the decorators who had come to paint the outside of her house and then they both realised the colour of her front door had been changed from green to yellow. Charlie had thought he was not going to Grannie's despite travelling the familiar journey. Only when Tibs, Grannie's cat, appeared in her doorway did Charlie understand that the house was the same, only the door colour had changed.

REFLECTIVE OASIS

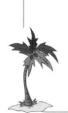

Can you think of an instance or situation where one detail had changed but the child with ASD had not recognised the whole picture?

How did you help the child to understand?

Did the child retain the memory of how it used to be?

Approaches to unwanted behaviours in young children

A popular mistake is to work to extinguish (remove) behaviour without planning to teach the child a more acceptable replacement. To punish and/or use aversive practices to respond to the behaviour will only teach the child fear, anxiety and a sense of discomfort. Although the outcome may be an element of conformity, the child will not have a reliable 'replacement' that gives the same message as the original behaviour. Often when we see a group of children conforming, we draw the conclusion that they do not have any challenging behaviours. We view conformity as a positive quality, indicating that everything is calm. But conformity can be a learned behaviour – if being quiet and sitting still is valued, the child with ASD may conform to avoid further stress.

Another popular mistake is to ignore the behaviour. This could amount to negligence and result in personal harm if the behaviour was self-stimulatory. We have to think of the safety and well-being of the other children in our care and do our best to protect them from unnecessary harm.

Behaviour as communication

Any form of extreme behaviour is 99 per cent a means of communicating something for the child with ASD. We need to pay attention to the message it conveys, or the behaviour will not be changed. What function is the behaviour serving for them. For example, do they get the object they want? Does it lessen demands made on them? Does it make people go away?

It will be important to:

- Collect the perceptions of important others – is the behaviour well established, does it occur with them, how do they respond?
- Reframe the way in which the behaviour is viewed by us or others. Is it viewed as deliberate or naughty?
- Think about how it could be shaped into something more acceptable and appropriate.
- A positive approach to the child and their behaviour is likely to achieve a better result and is more humane.
- Teach the child a socially acceptable way of achieving the same end result, e.g. pointing, use of pictures, a short phrase.

Strategies that react only to the behaviour (e.g. physical intervention) should be short-term. But also remember that difficult behaviour is not simple or speedy to change.

Look for the other reasons for the behaviour – could it be illness, fatigue, hunger?

Teach replacement skills. Help the young child to recognise when tension is mounting.

Help them to find ways in which they can effectively calm themselves – counting to 10, or red and green cards. (Holding up a red card indicates a high stress level; using a green card indicates that everything is fine.)

Finally, treat the behaviour as a form of communication – if the child could articulate what they felt at that particular point, what would they be saying?

Points to remember

- Behaviours may signal sensory overload or a situation of unbearable stress.
- Use the 'ASD lens' to examine the behaviour from the point of view of the child.
- The TEACCH approach can be used effectively at home and in an educational or care provision.
- Behaviour is often a means for communication – so look for the message!

9

Community involvement – helping young children to cope in the outside world

This chapter will look at ways in which the child can be helped to become more independent in their self-care skills, and more tolerant of family activities out in the local and wider community.

The young child with ASD may experience few challenges to their sense of safety and security when they are at home with a family who have often adapted their routines and lives to fit the child. Some families may have their lives governed by the wish to avoid an overreaction when carefully assembled toys in the hallway are dislodged or removed. The capacity to adapt family life to not upsetting the child with ASD is enormous. Little wonder that family wishes and routines get submerged in favour of maintaining the status quo.

There are children with ASD who feel comfortable and secure in their family home but who get distressed when they venture into the community. Two approaches have been developed for people with ASD that can be deployed within homes, families and the wider community.

The TEACCH approach

The Treatment and Education of Autistic and Communications handicapped Children (TEACCH) is an approach which utilises the strengths and emerging skills of the individual and focuses on the features of ASD to provide safety, predictability, structure and individualisation, delivering skills and tasks in a visually clear and logical way. Its originators claim a cradle-to-grave approach that will support the person with ASD through their lives. It requires no specialist resources, a small amount of training and can be adapted to the situation and the person (Schopler and Mesibov, 1995; Mesibov, Shea and Schopler, 2004; Mesibov and Howley, 2003; Wellman, 2005; **www.teacch.com**). Making everyday routines into a structure which can then be communicated visually to the young child with ASD, may assist in teaching many self-help/care skills. For instance, promoting independence in dressing order, hair combing, bathing, teeth cleaning and getting ready for bed, since all of these tasks are done in only one way. We do not put the toothpaste on the brush after we have finished brushing our teeth, nor do we ever put on socks before shoes, so these could be made into a pictorial schedule for the child to see what is going to happen, and to become involved in the routines.

Jamelia's get ready for bed list

1. Mummy baths Jamelia
2. Mummy dries Jamelia with the towel
3. Mummy puts on body cream
4. Jamelia puts on her PJs
5. Mummy and Jamelia go into Jamelia's room
6. Jamelia gets into bed
7. Mummy gives Jamelia a drink of water
8. Mummy says good night
9. Jamelia chooses a story
10. Daddy reads Jamelia one story
11. Daddy turns out the light
12. Daddy says good night
13. Jamelia goes to sleep

This visual schedule could be represented by objects of reference (reallife or miniature objects), by digital photographs of the child completing each stage, or by symbols or words, or any combination that works for the child.

Having the technology of digital photography or video cameras in our homes makes the reproduction of these simple activities in a visual format easy and personalised for each child. The photos can be affixed onto a card or wooden strip and then each stage's card can be removed once it is complete. There are countless instances of how visual formats have helped within the homes of young (and older) children, from showing the order and time of getting ready to go out to playgroup, to what is happening in the family on this particular morning. Once the child can trust the information on the schedule (because it has been proved to happen that way again and again), new and different activities can be introduced. Since things never quite go as planned, changes that are known about in advance can be put onto the schedule and the child will tolerate the circumstances better. If the child is not yet ready to understand photographs, then objects of reference can be used. Once the child can grasp the information conveyed by photos and objects of reference, it may be appropriate to introduce symbols or words with the pictures, which can build into using written phrases or sentences.

Wall (2004) gives many instances of how TEACCH can be used in an early years setting and then continued as the child enters school. Myles (2001) and Kluth (2003) have taken the strategies suggested by TEACCH to develop systems and structures within their teaching environments that use colour coding; equipment storage spaces; functionality of areas; schedules of activities; test reminders; and homework procedures. Myles also suggests compartmentalised backpacks for those who find it hard to organise themselves.

CASE STUDY

Although Narinder was about to start the Reception class at his local primary school, his parents had always struggled to teach him how to dress himself in the mornings. With a family of three other young children, the timetable for the day would begin with Mum or Dad rising at 5.30 to prepare all of the children for their daily activities. Mum or Dad would have to spend at least 45 minutes getting Narinder up and dressed, and this made his siblings feel that they were being neglected. Narinder had a great amount of dexterity with his special interests but appeared to be unable to roll up socks to put over his toes, or decide which of his legs to put in his trousers. With school starting in September, both parents were anxious that activities such as PE might highlight his lack of self-care skills. A nursery nurse suggested to them that using TEACCH schedule of visual information could help Narinder understand dressing skills. The nursery had had some success in getting Narinder to organise himself and stay on task by using TEACCH visual prompts.

Narinder's parents took digital photographs of each regularly-used item of Narinder's clothing. Then they mounted each digital image with Blu-tak onto a plain piece of card in order of dressing. So socks before shoes; vest before T-shirt; etc. Narinder's parents decided that they would teach waist-down dressing first, using the digital images in a sequential order, and pointing to each one as Narinder put them on. After several days they left his waist-down dressing schedule in his room and Narinder managed to get dressed by himself. The same approach was used with his upper torso and provided that his vest and tops were presented in the way to be put on (i.e. not inside out), he soon mastered those skills.

REFLECTIVE OASIS

Can you think of other self-care skills that follow a predictable and unvaried sequence?

How could the sequence of one of the above skills be presented to a child you know?

Would digital photos, objects of reference, symbols or words be the best medium to convey the visual order for the child you know?

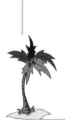

TEACCH can be used to great effect with some everyday, predictable skills. It can also be used out and about in the local community. Sometimes parents and carers do not make demands upon their child with ASD out in the community, and the child does not get exposed to typical family outings like weekly shopping for groceries, buying clothes, etc. Trips for family leisure activities may also be restricted because of strong opposition. Family holidays become out of the question. TEACCH can help prepare the child to anticipate what an outing is going to contain, and pictures of where you are going and what he is likely to see and do may actually help dispel a lot of the anxiety and stress. Often it is the 'not knowing' that causes the upset, but pictures and other visual markers will help to keep the situation calm.

Social stories

Social stories were developed by Carol Gray (1994) and they can be used to help people with ASD to learn how to handle situations, by giving explicit social information of what is happening. The story uses the situation as a focus and is written in either the first person or the third person (where the individual is referred to by name). There are specific sentences to use in each story:

- Descriptive: To define what happens – 'where', 'why' and 'what' statements. Occasionally it may be useful to use the word 'sometimes' to give flexibility.
- Directive: To state the desired response in a given situation and phrased in positive terms. It is better here to use terms like 'will try' rather than 'will do'.
- Perspective: To describe the behaviours, e.g. feelings, reactions, responses, of others involved in the situation.

Gray says that ideally the story should include between two and five descriptive and perspective statements for every directive statement, so that it does not become a list of instructions.

It is necessary to decide upon the behaviour (singular) that is causing problems and where it is most likely to occur. The story needs to be presented so that the child will understand – objects, photos, symbols or words can be used. It can also be illustrated with drawings. The story will need to be used on a regular basis and monitored carefully so as to gauge whether it has brought about a change in behaviour.

A sample social story

How to walk with Mum
When we go out to shops, Mum takes me in the car.
She parks the car in the car park by Tesco.
Mum likes me to hold her hand when we walk.
She says that will keep me safe.
She likes me to hold her hand when we get out of the car and walk over to the shopping centre.
When we get the shops I can walk by her side.
That will keep me safe.
I will try to hold her hand when we get out of the car and go to the shopping centre.

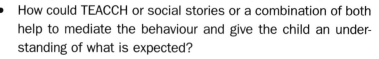

REFLECTIVE OASIS

- Can you define a particular social 'problem' that the child is struggling with?
- Is the problem with the child's social behaviour or with your feelings of embarrassment at how he is perceived by others?
- How could TEACCH or social stories or a combination of both help to mediate the behaviour and give the child an understanding of what is expected?

Jarvie (2005) used a combination of TEACCH visual scheduling and an accompanying social story (Gray, 2000) to prepare her son Keir, aged 5, for a four-week driving holiday for the whole family to Italy. Using photos and line drawings, she helped prepare Keir to tolerate a flight to Paris and a car journey to a mobile home in Italy. The length of journey time was represented by a car travelling along a Velcro road (manually moved) towards its destination. This success took place after a previous camping trip (without the visual detail) had had to be abandoned after two days.

Points to remember

- Often someone with ASD might feel comfortable at home in an adapted environment, but not have the same sense of security in a community setting.
- TEACCH is an approach which focuses on features of ASD and provides safety, predictability, structure and individualisation, delivering skills in a visually clear and logical way.
- TEACCH can give everyday routines a logical structure. Digital photography can help to personalise these schedules.
- Social stories have helped individuals handle situations that they might otherwise find difficult.
- Sometimes a combination of TEACCH and social stories helps to prepare for events outside the home such as a family holiday.

10

Alternative intervention and home-based programmes

This chapter looks at current approaches, interventions, programmes and common-sense strategies that are recommended for use with early years children. Specific (school) teaching or speech and language interventions are not included here, as the chapter aims to give impartial information to assist parents and practitioners in making informed choices.

Introduction

Sources of information on how best to help the person with ASD have reached millions in numbers with the advent of easy reference tools, such as the Google search engine. Treatments, interventions, approaches and strategies for helping young children with ASD can be easily accessed by a search engine. For parents who are trying to make sense of their child's condition and how best to help him/her, it can be a frustrating and misleading medium, making them very vulnerable. Key elements found to be present in effective intervention programmes were identified by Dawson and Osterling (1997) as:

- a focus on specific skills that the child learns
- a structured environment that provides opportunities to transfer skills and knowledge (generalisation)

- predictability and routine-based
- involves the whole family.

When considering any approach or intervention, it is always worth asking the following questions:

- In what ways does the approach address all three areas of the triad of impairments?
- What are the claims of the approach and where is the evidence to back these up?
- What are the time- and people-commitments?
- Is it legal, respectful and accepting of the person with ASD?
- Does it seek to change them into a quasi-neurotypical?

Keyhole Project (2003) and Rainbow Resource Kit

The Keyhole Project (PAPA, 2003) was undertaken in recognition of the increasing numbers of children being diagnosed with ASD in Northern Ireland under the age of 4. The Project aimed to make recommendations to parents on 'an holistic approach to interventions' for children aged between 2 and 4. The Project was evaluated independently by the University of Ulster. The researchers interviewed the key stakeholders in early intervention: parents and carers; home visiting services; pre-school providers; and parent support groups, obtaining qualitative and qualitative data from each sub-group. They completed interviews with 72 families; offered home-based intervention with 24 families and did a follow-up evaluation of this work; surveyed 38 pre-school providers and trained 64 members of staff; collated 68 questionnaire responses from their membership; facilitated 15 mothers in a support meeting; and developed their own training materials.

Their examination of home-based programme provision was conducted over 12 months and they worked with families of children with a diagnosis of ASD who were under the age of 4 and not attending a pre-school service. The programme was delivered in three stages:

- assessment and information-gathering
- intensive input using TEACCH
- training parents in language and communication style and input
- using PECS to develop expression and communicative intent
- forward planning of smooth transition to pre-school placement
- monthly follow-up.

All 20 children showed gains in communication, daily living skills and socialisation. There were no perceived gains in motor skills. Some 95 per cent of families reported benefits from receiving the programme and consequently fewer perceived problems with their child's behaviour, play and language skills.

The Keyhole Project report makes a number of recommendations:

- that home-based intervention should be made available to parents/carers as part of the assessment and diagnostic process, and be delivered by health trust personnel
- the form and content of home-based programmes should address the individual needs of the child and the circumstances of the family
- a named person (delivering the home-based programme) should act as the conduit to other professionals
- training for parents and the professionals involved in delivering a home-based programme should be available and developmental.

PAPA as a parent-led organisation has developed a number of initiatives to address these recommendations including their six ACCESS workshops for parents/carers, Keyhole Autism Training in collaboration with Barnardos and NIPPA (Northern Ireland Preschool Playgroups Association), and the Rainbow Resource Kit (**www.autismni.org**).

Applied behaviour analysis (ABA – Lovaas programmes)

Behavioural methods have been used in the education and behaviour-training of children with special educational needs (SEN) from the late 1960s. Educational and clinical psychologists have used techniques of reinforcing (rewarding) desired behaviours and using deterrents to non-acceptable behaviours for many decades (Kiernan et al., 1978). Over time, the strategies have been modified and adapted, with deterrents such as physical punishment no longer recognised as appropriate or, in some cases, legal. Ivar Lovaas, a Norwegian practising in America, has taken the basis of applied behaviour analysis and discrete trial learning (Lovaas, 1981) to modify the behaviours exhibited by children with ASD. The hypothesis is that all human behaviour is learned and that it is governed by both its triggers and consequences.

Between 1970 and 1984, Lovaas and his colleagues ran the Young Autism Project with a group of 59 children with ASD, with trained therapists and parents using behavioural techniques in a home-based programme. The recommended timing for the intervention is up to 40 hours per week for around 24 months, using family members and supervised volunteers. Each session lasts two to three hours, and the child is taken through a series of repertoires (drills) of 10–15 minutes each. The child has a break of up to five minutes between changes in tasks. The Early Intensive Behavioural Intervention (EIBI) component is recommended for children between the ages of 2 and 4, taking part in one-to-one intensive work for 20–30 hours per week (**www.lovaas.com**).

The positive gains from the programme may be as a result of:

high intensity of adult support, one-to-one or sometimes two-to-one
high level of intervention time (up to 40 hours)
concerted period of time (up to three years)
standardised approach
scripted adult responses for continuity
lack of reaction to unwanted behaviours (other than re-direction or distraction).

Recent research undertaken by Professor Phil Reed and associates has compared the use of ABA with other interventions (Portage or attendance at special nursery) (Reed, Osborne and Corness, 2006). The authors point out that the measures used in the original study by Lovaas and his associates (1987) had some potential problems in its construction, and different measures were used, pre- and post-intervention. Other criticisms (Shea, 2004) point to lack of equivalence in groups of children studied; possibility of other approaches being used at the same time; and lack of data on how the approach was followed. The research by Reed et al. (2006) concentrated on using ABA in two different time intensities (30 hours per week and 12 hours per week). The 30 hours per week intensity showed bigger gains in standard tests, but higher-intensity gains were not in direct proportion to the lower-intensity programme (i.e. they were not 2.5 times better). Their work looking at predictors of school successes (Reed, Osborne and Waddington, 2006) makes tentative conclusions that children with ASD who have taken part in ABA, exhibit fewer behavioural problems at school, but are less socialised than those who had been to special nursery.

The Lovaas ABA approach has many strong advocates within the UK (Bibby et al., 2002; PEACH, **www.peach.uk.com**) and parents receive a high level of support and contact with trained therapists who are working with their child.

Recent research by Shea (2004) points out that attempts to replicate the outcomes of the original research by Lovaas and associates have not been able to achieve the same successes. The results of many replication studies are available only on the Internet and have not received the scrutiny and academic rigour of being submitted for journal publication.

Option approach (Son-Rise programme)

This home-based programme was developed in Massachusetts, USA by parents (the Kaufmans) who had a young child with ASD. Their son, Raun, is now in his 30s and he, along with his parents and sister, offer training on their Son-Rise programme. The Kaufmans claim that their work with their son has helped him to recover from his ASD. Their work has been the subject of a BBC *QED* programme (BBC, 1996) which followed a family from the West Midlands who took their son to the Option Institute (Kaufman, 1976, 1994; **www.option.org**).

The key features of this approach are that it is child-centred, 'to love is to be happy with', and home-based, preferably with a 'den' or specially created environment (playroom) for the child. The room needs to be distraction-free and provide safety and security.

Using the 'three Es' – excitement, enthusiasm and energy – the adults take the lead from the child, without direction or instruction, making interactions accepting and non-confrontational. Parents/caregivers are seen as the child's most important resource.

The programme focuses on developing a relationship with the child, with unconditional acceptance and respect, valuing what they do and making the child feel at ease. The aim is to enter the child's world, rather than expect them to join ours: 'They show us the way in and we show them the way out' (Kaufman, 2002). The response of adults is similar to Intensive Interaction (Nind and Hewett, 1994) in building on the child' attempts to communicate and interact, by responding to them with delight in their responses. Like the Hanen approach (see p. 68), the involvement, training and follow-up of parents/caregivers gives them the confidence and motivation to ensure progress. As part of the training, parents are videoed and then the film is played back, with professional therapists in attendance to talk through what they observe and how to shape the parents' and the child's responses.

Greenspan Floor Time

The Greenspan approach (or Floor Time model) focuses on a developmental model. Greenspan believes that most interventions target the areas that have been the subject of initial observation during diagnosis – motor, sensory, behaviour, language and communication, instead of looking at a broader overview of challenges to the child (Greenspan and Weider, 2006 **www. stanleygreenspan.com**).

Greenspan states that each child will bring physical differences, while each PCG will brings the wider arena of family life and environment and their own interactive style. The child's developmental progression is not determined by physical differences, nor is it due to the way in which the child is cared for, the environment or family and cultural influences. Rather, it develops over time in its own specific context. He believes that there cannot be a 'one size fits all' approach, and any approach must build on the child–family relationship rather than the child–professional relationship.

Greenspan shows developmental stages of relating and communicating as a way to gauge where the child is functioning.

For example:

At birth to 8 months: Does the baby smile joyfully in response to vocalisation and facial expression?
At 6 to 18 months: How does the child combine gestures and words to communicate?
At 18 to 36 months: How does the chid use pretend play to communicate emotional themes such as curiosity, independence and rejection?
At 36 to 60 months: How does the child control impulses and stabilise moods?

(Taken from **www.coping.org/earlyin/floortm.htm** accessed 29/01/04)

From these specific questions, one can see that some of the differences evident in the development of a young child with ASD are picked up on. Greenspan then takes the parent/practitioner through to looking at goal behaviours, e.g. taking initiative, sequencing longer and more complex actions and communications, and mapping these onto floor time activities that can work towards the attainment of the goal.

Greenspan's Floor Time is broken down into five steps:

- taking time to observe and notice the child's responses and emotions
- opening up a 'circle of communication', where interactions can be built from

- using the child's lead and becoming a 'supportive partner'
- beginning to expand and extend the nature of the interactions
- allowing the child to complete the 'circle' by moving through a range of interactions.

The approach, like others, encourages parents and practitioners to accept the child where they are, and to show respect for them by not changing how they interact or teaching them how to behave. Their prompts for adults to self-check on whether they are a 'good floor-timer' act as a reminder, for example:

Do I use a calm voice?
Are my actions non-intrusive?
Do I observe the child's style of relating?

Their suggestions for useful resources to help support floor time activities are the types of toys and equipment that most households with children would possess, e.g. road signs, doctor's kit, doll's bed, plastic farm animals. Each set of resources is grouped under its potential usefulness to initiate specific interactions like fantasy play, nurturing and empathy activities, construction play.

Intensive interaction

This approach was originally developed in an adult hospital provision – Harperbury Hospital – by Nind and Hewett for people with severe learning disabilities (SLD), who did not have functional communication systems (Hewett and Nind,1998; Nind and Hewett, 1994; **www.intensiveinteraction. co.uk**). Although they did not necessarily have a diagnosis of ASD, their behaviours and characteristics mirrored many features associated with ASD. The approach bases its strategies on early communication interaction between caregivers and very young children. The PCG uses imitation, exaggeration and acting on every move, non-verbal gesture or vocalisation, as if it is an attempt to communicate.

Using such strategies to engage with the individual with ASD, an imitation 'game' can be established. Moving on, opportunities to alter and extend the child's responses will be given, always respecting the responses of the child if they wish to stop. The aim is to engage and prolong interactions by building up visual attention and a shared interaction, thus providing a scaffold for establishing a repertoire of enjoyable experiences.

Nind and Hewett (1994) note progress in child sociability, communicative intent and willingness to participate, where previously they had appeared 'unavailable' to such interactions. Parents and caregivers use their instincts and close knowledge of the child to build up a series of mutually enjoyable games, which brings them closer together. The approach can be used with people with ASD at any age. However, the older the individual is, the higher the reticence and potential embarrassment of the parent/practitioner in engaging in what could be misinterpreted by others as 'babying'.

The Hanen approach

The Hanen approach uses strategies, which, as one parent says, 'are the opposite of what you might naturally do when there is a breakdown in communication' (Batts, 2000). Instead of telling the child what to do, the Hanen approach advocates working around the resistance or reluctance of the child to communicate (Sussman, 1999). This can give the child the pleasure and fun of communicating, rather than lead to conflict and/or rejection.

By using the 'three As', we can:

Adapt our communicative attempts to what the child is interested in
Add by elaborating on the communicative attempts of the child
Allow them to take the lead.

Batts (2000) used this approach with her partially hearing sons and became an advocate of the approach with them, and then in her professional work as a paediatric nurse with children with ASD.

The Hanen Centre, based in Toronto, Canada, was established in 1977 and has published guidebooks and programmes aimed at helping parents and professionals to encourage young children and non-communicating adults to have a functional system of communication (**www.hanen.org**). Their 'More than words' programme was devised to help parents help their young child with ASD. This programme draws on specific strategies for those with ASD, in a structured environment that encourages communication, following the child's lead and building upon their attempts at communication. One simple idea is not to make everything easily accessible for the child, but putting preferred objects just out of reach so that communication is prompted. What people with ASD often lack is the need to communicate if everything is anticipated and made accessible for them.

The programme has the aim to empower parents, caregivers and family members to offer communicative experiences to the person with ASD in a non-threatening and nurturing way. In keeping with other successful approaches (Jordan, Jones and Murray, 1998), the involvement and skilling-up of parents and families to feel confident in their exchanges with the child, is the key to ensuring progress and success.

The Hanen Centre has produced the *Learning Language and Loving It* programme for use by practitioners in pre-school settings.

The EarlyBird programme

In 1997, the National Autistic Society set up the EarlyBird programme as a pilot project (Shields, 1999, 2000). Since the pilot project, the EarlyBird programme is now offered via voluntary organisations, such as parent-led societies, LEA provisions and other agencies. It aims to support parents of young children with ASD, post-diagnosis and before they start an educational placement. It is a three-month programme which was designed for pre-school children and their parents. The programme takes six families at a time and they meet on a weekly basis. Group training sessions are offered alongside home visits, where a practitioner works with the parent/carer together with the child. Video recording is made for feedback purposes to help parents practise what they have learned.

EarlyBird says its three main targets are

- to help parents understand the condition of ASD
- to teach and practise skills that will help develop communication
- to assist parent/carers to analyse and manage their child's behaviour.

The EarlyBird Programme also encompasses aspects of PECS (Bondy and Frost, 1994), SPELL (Siddles et al., 1997) and TEACCH (Schopler and Mesibov, 1995). Handouts and information from each session are compiled into a handbook and parent/carers also have homework tasks. Training is available for professionals with experience of ASD for licensed use of the package.

The Maytree Autistic Programme run at a nursery school in south London (Smith, 2005) uses the principles of EarlyBird to support parents/carers with information and advice. They take the approach to another level by making their contact with and support of parents last the duration of the placement at nursery via a dedicated outreach worker, who will help parent and child anticipate and prepare for transition into primary schooling. The nursery setting itself uses visual approaches, anticipation, preparation and rehearsal, extra staff support at social times and the opportunity to work in a visually screened space to enable the young child with ASD cope with what is often a busy and confusing environment.

Dalton and Tasker (2002) evaluated the running of four EarlyBird training programmes by their Coventry Autism Support Service, which has six licensed EarlyBird trainers. They felt that timing and fitting in training and practice sessions could be a pressure, as could the amount of information given to parents at each session. Some parents were wary of videoing their child in the home and the programme evaluation via long questionnaires could be offputting to parents.

A study of these parents' qualitative responses undertaken by Morris (2002) picks out few gains in the area of communication reported by parents of their children, but much greater gains in joint attention, play and social activities. Other reported gains were parents being more patient and waiting for their child to respond, more relaxed interactions with their child, and altered perception of the child's strengths. However, Morris warns that follow-up of the programme is hard to arrange, as trainers move on to the next cohort of parents. Sometimes trained parents would benefit from 'top-up sessions' to keep their skills honed and their confidence levels high.

The Portage programme

The Portage programme was designed to support pre-school children with special needs, and is on offer around the UK, usually by an LEA pre-school team. The Portage worker will work on specific targets and skills with the child and parents via weekly or fortnightly home visits (Bluma et al., 1976; Cameron, 1986). The National Portage Association has been involved in developing and evaluating materials specifically for use with children with social and communication difficulties, including those with an ASD (**www.portage. org.uk**).

Recent comparative research undertaken by Reed, Osborne and Corness (2006) looked at the effectiveness of the Portage programme against applied behaviour analysis (Lovaas, 1981, 1987) and attendance at a special nursery. The children studied were aged between 2.6 and 4 years old, and were studied over nine months of intervention/attendance. All children in the research (n=48) showed measurable developmental gains, although the 16 in the Portage programme did not match the other two approaches in terms of academic progress (ABA) or social skills and adaptive behaviours (special nursery).

The Hampshire Outline for Meeting the Needs of under-5s on the Autistic Spectrum (THOMAS) approach

The THOMAS approach was initially a booklet produced by a working party of early years professionals within one local authority (Hampshire) (**www.Hants.gov.uk/tc/inclusion/thomassummary.html**). The booklet aimed to help providers feel skilled and confident in their work with young children with ASD, and could also be given to parents on request. This was followed by the provision of four-day training sessions for professionals and parents, with the invitation being extended other key carers (grandparents) and associated professionals (SALTs and other therapists). A specialised TOP (THOMAS Outreach Project) service was established, which followed up children in the home or in educational placements. An evaluative study, undertaken by Smith and McSpadden (2002), charts the evolution and development of a very comprehensive local authority response to parents/carers of young children with or awaiting a diagnosis of ASD.

Interventions by the TOP workers show, with as little as three months' worth of interventions (of eight hours per week), marked gains in social interaction, language and communication, play and tolerance levels, as well as motor skills, behaviours conducive to learning and pre-literacy and numeracy skills. All showed evidence of increase over baseline assessments. Qualitative responses by parents/carers highlight new confidence in their own skills and enjoyment of their child.

Summary

Each of the approaches mentioned has had their champions and detractors. Some bear a striking similarity to each other, and some are well suited to be used together. There is much more to do in terms of independent and impartial evaluation of why an approach works. There is no single approach that will work with all individuals with ASD and, at the time of writing, few seem to address the population of people with ASD and a high IQ. Other books in this series deal with educational strategies (Plimley and Bowen, 2006a) but many of those mentioned in this chapter can be transferred from home to school.

REFLECTIVE OASIS

Consider two or three of the approaches mentioned in this chapter. What would you need to do to instigate the approach in your home or setting?

Does the approach feel comfortable for you to be involved in as an adult?

How might a child with ASD that you know react and respond to the approach?

Points to remember

- A range of approaches and strategies exists with the aim of meeting the needs of children with ASD.
- Some approaches are compatible and can therefore be used together.
- Decisions to use an approach must be based on individual need – every child is unique. There is no 'one size fits all'.

11

Transition planning

This chapter discusses the strategies that might be adopted to make the transition from one service to another as stress-free as possible for the young child with ASD. It makes suggestions as to who might be involved in the process and how the environment and curriculum might need to change to accommodate individual needs. It focuses on the move from pre-school settings into school.

Pre-school provision

Wall (2004) states that early years provision now includes a variety of services providers. In the statutory system, these include primary schools, nursery schools, day nurseries and home-based support, and in the private sector, these can include childminders, private nurseries and nannies or au pairs. Some children may have attended groups organised by the voluntary sector such as pre-school play groups. The child will eventually move from settings provided by health, social services, the private sector or the voluntary, into a mainstream or special school environment.

Forward planning

Moving to a new environment can give rise to fear and trauma for many children. Some children may have spent very little time away from a parent or a childminder and so the onset of the separation process for time at another setting will need careful forward planning.

For the young child with ASD, the sooner the preparation for the newer environment can take place, the better. New staff will need to become familiar with the child's needs, prior to placement. It is important that new staff learn to draw on the knowledge of those who know the child well such as parents/carers, siblings, health professionals and staff from other settings, where relevant.

Staff should consider continuity – how can things that are working well in one environment be transferred to another? The setting SENCo should be able to provide information and suggestions for individual play plans, areas of strength and behaviour management strategies.

Working with parents/carers

Bache et al. (2004) stress the importance of new staff meeting parents/carers. They suggest that answers to the following basic questions can be very useful in assisting forward planning:

What strategies and language is the child familiar with at home?

Would this be appropriate to use in the new setting?

Does the child have particular sensitivities such as food, touch, smell, sleep difficulties?

How did the child settle into other settings?

Were any particular strategies required that could support the move?

Useful meetings

PAPA (2003) in the *ASD Teacher's Toolkit* suggests that the following three types of meetings can be useful in planning the move from pre-school to school setting.

1. Getting to know pupils

A general meeting should be held of parents, SENCo, special educational needs teaching assistants, the class teacher, the head teacher and relevant health professionals. This meeting could also include staff from the pre-school setting. The purpose of the meeting is to get a general overview of the child's abilities, strengths and needs.

2. School staff

The special needs teacher/SENCo, class teacher and head teacher meet to review information from the first meeting and available material. This group can draw up a short-term plan or IEP outlining for example:

- learning goals for the child
- amount of time spent in school (less than other pupils initially if required)
- time in resources
- manner in which breaks and lunchtimes should be managed
- role of classroom assistant
- details of any other changes required.

3. Parents and school staff

A meeting between school staff and parents should be arranged to discuss any plans made by the school. A definite date should be given for a follow-up meeting, for example in one month.

PAPA states that when the plan is implemented, the child should settle in with fewer problems because time has been taken to think about his/her needs. Also when the school staff are more familiar with the pupil's needs, the year's programme can be discussed.

CASE STUDY

The SENCo of an infants' school works closely with social services and health professionals. When a young child in her area is identified as having SEN she liaises closely with parents and the staff in playgroup to make preparations for the move to nursery class. She concentrates on the self-help skills and social skills that may need to be addressed before the child goes to school. An IEP is drawn up and carefully monitored by all involved.

The SENCo also meets with parents/carers and has made a range of leaflets and pamphlets that will help them to work with their child at home and understand the school system more fully. She recognises that some parents may wish to discuss this information with her in an informal way.

(With thanks to Hafod Y Wern Infants, Wrexham)

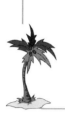

REFLECTIVE OASIS

What procedures do you have in place to ensure the smooth transition between settings?
How many people do you involve in this process?
How do you draw up an individual plan for the child and with whom?

Implications for teaching the Foundation Stage

The Foundation Stage (QCA/DfEE, 2000) was introduced in England and provides a framework for the provision of education across a range of early years settings, and is for children aged 3 to the end of Reception. It is designed to prepare children for Key Stage 1 and is in line with the National Curriculum. All children follow a curriculum which helps them make progress towards Early Learning Goals. At the end of the Stage some children will have achieved all the goals, while others will still be working towards them. The Foundation Phase has also been piloted in Wales (WAG, 2006b).

In England, six areas of learning are identified:

- personal, social and emotional development
- communication, language and literacy
- mathematical development
- knowledge and understanding of the world
- physical development
- creative development.

In Scotland (Scottish CCC,1999) the same areas of learning are addressed for this age group of children. In Wales, there is an additional area – bilingualism and multicultural understanding. In Northern Ireland (DENI, 1997), 'Early experiences in science and technology' is an additional area of learning, but the system has recently undergone a major review (DENI, 2006). All plans stress the importance of working closely with parents and carers.

Cumine et al. (2000) have examined the areas of learning identified in England, in relation to young children with ASD. They have recommended a number of strategies that would assist in the learning process. Such strategies would need careful consideration in the transition process.

Personal, social and emotional development

Cumine et al. argue that attention needs to be given to such issues as establishing relationships, co-operating in pairs, small groups and whole-class activities and understanding feelings. Opportunities to make choices and participate in challenging activities should also be provided.

Communication, language and literacy

Areas for consideration include helping the child to understand what communication involves and giving him/her the verbal and non-verbal strategies. Language can be linked to certain songs and rhymes, but also to real-life experiences and a range of social situations.

Mathematical development

The focus could be on extending areas of strength (e.g. manipulation of shapes) and using mathematical concepts in real-life situations and activities.

Physical development

Attention should be given to issues such as health and safety, team building and overcoming any anxieties.

Knowledge and understanding of the world

Children need to be encouraged to draw upon their past experiences to predict, problem-solve and make choices. First-hand experiences help them to reflect upon their actions and the part they have to play in such activities.

Creative development

Young children must be given the opportunity to develop their creative skills. Pretend-play skills may well be limited, so activities using real and concrete objects and situations may need to be a starting point. Sensory preferences can motivate children to explore their environment, and the child should be encouraged to make connections between past and present activities. Some youngsters will find certain things intolerable, e.g. sand, clay, paint.

CASE STUDY

Jessie loved to play with brightly coloured metallic shapes. She was encouraged to use this interest in a constructive way by sitting at the side of an adult and using the shapes to copy a sequence (maths). She was also encouraged to ask for 'her' shapes using picture symbols (language and communication). She was given the shapes to play with as a reward especially after an activity which she had found challenging (PSE).

REFLECTIVE OASIS

Choose one area of learning. How might you use a child's special interest to maximise learning potential in this particular area?

Creating the right environment

Early years settings are usually very busy places. There is noise, much to see, plenty of movement. and lots of surprises. For the young child with ASD, who finds it difficult to make sense of the world, this can cause a great deal of anxiety. Little things might make them behave in an inappropriate way, e.g. the smell of disinfectant in the toilet, the feel of a label on the back of a painting apron, or proximity of other children during story time. It is important for staff in early years settings to work with parents/carers to build up a profile of the child's likes and dislikes so that stressful situations can be avoided.

Making the best use of space

General strategies can be employed to make life more tolerable. For example:

How is the space utilised in terms of furniture and equipment?
Is the room organised in such a way that children know what is expected of them and where?

Visual clues make it clear that different areas are for different activities. Resources for the activity should be labelled and colour-coded using the same visual clue.

Sometimes it is difficult for children to know where to sit, when there is so much choice, so labelling chairs and tables is also useful and avoids disruption. Think about the light, heating and noise levels in the room. Consider health and safety issues too – many youngsters with ASD will take flight when anxiety levels rise.

Structuring the day

Visual timetables are important to help a child know what is happening throughout the day. It is important to build in times when the child can take some time out from the rest of the group and have a balance between potentially stressful times and stress-free times. For example, activities that are socially demanding need to be balanced with times to play alone with a favourite toy or object. Pay particular attention to lunch times and break times, which can be particularly stressful. Cards with symbols, photographs or drawings can be used and attached to a board using Velcro. Timetables can run from right to left or from top to bottom, and children can take responsibility for taking the card down once the activity has ended. It is important for an adult to run through the timetable at the start of the day. Knowing when one activity ends and the next begins can be difficult for young children. Useful strategies include:

- traffic light system – green for go, amber meaning start putting things away, and red for stop
- picture symbols on a Velcro strip taking children through each step of the task
- start and finish boxes
- egg timers
- clocks.

Providing a 'safe haven'

Early years settings can often be brightly decorated. Sometimes this can be overpowering for the young child with ASD. Set aside a quiet corner of the room that can be used as a 'safe haven' and for one-to-one teaching. If space is a problem, a table facing a bare wall or a bean bag chair in the corner of the room may suffice.

Using the right language

The language of the learning environment needs to be kept simple and explicit. For example, do not speak as if you are offering choices: 'Shall we go and play in the sand now?' or use abstract phrases such as 'Line up' or 'Make a circle'. If you want the child with ASD to attend, always use his/her name first. Try not to use open-ended questions, e.g. 'What do you want to drink?' It is better to say 'Juice or water?' and show visual symbols as a prompt. Always give the child the opportunity and time to process language.

Most young children with ASD are unlikely to respond to group instructions. Using picture symbols will help the child with little language to communicate needs and preferences. Choice boards are a good way of doing this. A card with the words 'I want' can be placed at the top of the board, with picture symbols or photographs of the choices available underneath.

The transition from a school environment to the home

In some circumstances parents make the decision to remove their child from school and educate them at home. Holland (2005) made such a decision. She argues that there still needs to be a clear difference between the home environment and the teaching environment. She made her garage into a school room and made sure there was a clear structure to the teaching day.

REFLECTIVE OASIS

How can you make your setting more 'ASD friendly'?

Points to remember

- Plan well in advance with parents and professionals.
- Differentiation of the curriculum.
- Modify the environment to relieve stress and maximise learning potential.
- Give the day structure and routine.
- Language and communication.

References

ACCAC (2002) *A Focus on Achievement: Guidance on Including Pupils with Additional Needs in Whole School Target Setting.* Birmingham: ACCAC

ACCAC (2004) *The Foundation Phase in Wales: A Draft Framework for Children's Learning.* Cardiff: National Assembly for Wales

American Psychiatric Association (1994) *Diagnostic and Statistical Manual of Mental Health version IV.* Washington, DC: American Psychiatric Association

Attfield, E. and Morgan, H. (2006) *Living with Autistic Spectrum Disorders.* London: Sage/Paul Chapman Publications

Audit Commission (2002) *Policy Focus: Statutory Assessment and Statements of SEN: in need of review?* Pontypool: MWL Print Group

Bache, K., Daniels, E., Hewison, S. and Young, P. (2004) *Guidelines for Working with Children with ASD at Foundation Stage and KS1.* **www.southglos.gov.uk**

Baron-Cohen, S., Allen, J. and Gillberg, C. (1992) Can autism be detected at 18 months? The needle, the haystack and the CHAT. *British Journal of Psychiatry, 161,* 839–843

Batts, S. (2000) *More than words can say.* http://community.nursingspectrum.com (accessed 01/06/06)

Bibby, P., Eikseth, S., Martin, N.T., Mudford, O.C. and Reeves, D. (2002) Progress and outcomes for children with Autism receiving parent-managed intensive interventions. *Research in Developmental disabilities, 23, 81–104*

Bleach, F. (2001) *Everybody is Different: A Book for Young People Who Have Brothers or Sisters with Autism.* London: NAS Publications

Bluma, S.M., Shearer, J., Frohman, A.H. and Hilliard, J.M. (1976) *Portage Guide to Early Education.* Windsor: Cooperative Educational Service Agency

Bogdashina, O. (2003) *Sensory Perceptual Issues in Autism and Asperger Syndrome. Different Sensory Experiences Different Perceptual Worlds.* London: Jessica Kingsley

Bondy, A. and Frost, L. (1994) The Delaware autistic program, in S.L. Harris and J.S. Handleman (eds) *Preschool Education Programs for Children with Autism.* Austin, Texas: Pro-Ed

British Broadcasting Corporation (1996) *QED* programme on the Option approach, shown 30 May

Cameron, R.J. (1986) *Portage: Preschoolers, Parents and Professionals: Ten Years of Achievement in the UK.* Windsor: NFER-Nelson

Corea, I. (2003) BME Communities – Autism and Asperger syndrome. **http://autism-ethnic-uk.tripod.com**

Cumine, V., Leach, J. and Stevenson, G. (1998) *Asperger Syndrome: A Practical Guide for Teachers.* London: David Fulton

Cumine, V., Leach, J. and Stevenson, G. (2000) *Autism in the Early Years.* London: David Fulton

Dalton, H. and Tasker, J. (2002) NAS EarlyBird programme: a local authority perspective. *Good Autism Practice Journal. Early Intervention Edition.* Kidderminster: BILD

Davis, J. (1994a) *Able Autistic Children: A Booklet for Brothers and Sisters.* Nottingham: Early Years Diagnostic Centre

Davis, J. (1994b) *Children with Autism: A Booklet for Brothers and Sisters.* Nottingham: Early Years Diagnostic Centre

Dawson, G. and Osterling, J. (1997) Early intervention in autism, in Guralnick, M. (ed.) *The Effectiveness of Early Intervention.* Baltimore, MD: Brookes

De Clercq, H. (2001) Talk given by Hilda de Clercq to staff at Coddington Court school, Herefordshire

Department of Education and Employment (1996) *Education Act.* London: HMSO

Department for Education and Skills (DfES) (2001) *Special Educational Needs and Disability Act (SENDA).* London: HMSO

Department for Education and Skills (DfES) (2002a) *Autistic Spectrum Disorders: Good Practice Guidance.* Nottingham: DfES

ASD Good Practice Guidance – Early Years Examples **www.teachernet.gov.uk**

Department for Education and Skills (DfES) (2002b) *The SEN Code of Practice.* London: HMSO

Department for Education and Skills (DfES) (2003) *Every Child Matters.* London: HMSO **www.everychildmatters.gov.uk/multiagencyworking**

Department for Education and Skills (DfES) (2004) *Children Act.* London: HMSO

Department of Work and Pensions (1995) *The Disability Discrimination Act.* London: HMSO

Department of Education Northern Ireland (DENI) (1997) *Curricular Guidance.* Bangor, Co Down: Department of Education Northern Ireland

Department of Education Northern Ireland (DENI) (2005a) *Special educational needs and disability order (SENDO).* **www.deni.gov.uk/index/7special_educational_needs_pg/ special_needs-legislation_pg/special_educational_needs_-_legislation_sendo_pg.htm**

Department of Education Northern Ireland (DENI) (2005b) *Supplement to the Code of Practice on Identification and Assessment of Special Educational Need.* Bangor, Co Down: Department of Education Northern Ireland

Department of Education Northern Ireland (DENI) (2006) *Review of Pre-school Education in Northern Ireland.* Bangor, Co Down: Department of Education Northern Ireland

Dickinson, P. and Hannah, E. (1998) *It Can Get Better – Dealing with Common Behaviour Problems in Young Autistic Children.* London: NAS

DiLavore, P., Lord, C. and Rutter, M. (1995) Pre-Linguistic Autism Diagnostic Observation Schedule (PL/ADOS). *Journal of Autism and Developmental Disorders,* 25, 355–379

Estyn (2004) *Best Practice in the Development of Statements of Special Educational Needs and the Delivery by Schools of the Action Agreed.* Cardiff: Crown Copyright

Filipek, P.A., Accardo, P. J., Baranek, G.T., Cook, E.H., Dawson, G., Gordon, B., Gravel, H., Johnson, C.P., Kallen, R.J., Levy, S.E., Minshew, N.J., Ozonoff, S., Prizant, B.M., Rapin, I.,

Rogers, S.J., Stone, W.L., Teplin, S.W., Tuchman, R.F. and Volkmar, F.R. (1999) The screening and diagnosis of autism spectrum disorders. *Journal of Autism and Developmental Disorders*, 29, 437–482

Frith, U. (1989) *Autism: Explaining the Enigma*. Oxford: Blackwell

Gillberg, C. (1989) Asperger's syndrome in 23 Swedish children. *Developmental medicine and child neurology, 31, 520–531*

Gillberg, C. (1991) The Emmanuel Miller Memorial lecture 1991: Autism and autistic-like conditions. *Journal of Child Psychology and Psychiatry,* 33, 813–842

Gillberg, C., Gillberg, C., Rastam, M. and Wentz, E. (2001) The Asperger syndrome (and high-functioning autism) diagnostic interview (ASDI): a preliminary study of a new structured clinical interview. *Autism,* 5, 57–66

Gordon Smith, P. (2005) A map for families with autistic children. *Early Education,* Spring, 3–5

Gorrod, L. (1997) *My Brother is Different: A Book for Young Children Who Have Brothers and Sisters with Autism.* London, NAS Publications

Gray, A.C. (1994) *Social Stories.* Arlington: Future Horizons

Gray, A.C. (2000) *The New Social story book: illustrated edition.* Arlington, TX: Future Horizons

Greenspan, S. and Wieder, S. (2006) *Engaging Autism: Using the Floortime approach to Help Children Relate, Communicate and Think.* New York: Di Capo Press

Guralnick, M. (ed.) (1997) *The Effectiveness of Early Intervention.* Baltimore, MD: Brookes

Hewett, D. and Nind, M. (eds) (1998) *Interaction in Action.* London: David Fulton

Holland, O. (2005) *Teaching at Home.* London: Jessica Kingsley

Jackson, L. (2002) *Freaks, Geeks and Asperger Syndrome.* London: Jessica Kingsley

Jarvie, L. (2005) Supporting my son on our trip to Italy. *Good Autism Practice Journal,* 6(1), 35–37

Jordan, R.R. (1999) *Autistic Spectrum Disorders – An Introductory Handbook for Practitioners.* London: David Fulton

Jordan, R., Jones, G. and Murray, D. (1998) *Educational interventions for children with autism: a literature review of recent and current research, Report 77.* Sudbury: DfEE

Kaufman, B.N. (1976) *To Love is to be Happy With.* London: Souvenir Press

Kaufman, B.N. (1994) *Son Rise the Miracle Continues.* New York: Warner

Kaufman, R.K. (2002) Building the bridges: strategies for reaching our children. *Good Autism Practice Journal. Early Years Edition*

Kiernan, C., Jordan, R. and Saunders, C.A. (1978) *Starting Off.* London: Souvenir Press.

Kluth, P. (2003) *You're Gonna Love this Kid.* London: Jessica Kingsley

Lacey, P. (2001) *Support Partnerships: Collaboration in Action.* London: David Fulton

Le Breton, M. (2001) *Diet Intervention and Autism : Implementing the Gluten Free and Casein Free Diet for Autistic Children and Adults – A Practical Guide for Parents.* London: Jessica Kingsley

Lord, C., Rutter, M., Goode, S., Heemsbergen, J., Jordan, H., Mawhood, L. and Schopler E. (1989) Autism Diagnostic Observation Schedule – ADOS – a standardised observation of communication and behaviour. *Journal of Autism and Developmental disorders,* 19, 185–212

Lord, C., Rutter, M. and Le Couteur, A. (1994) Autism Diagnostic Interview – Revised: a revised version of a diagnostic interview for care-givers of individuals with possible pervasive developmental disorders. *Journal of Autism and Developmental Disorders,* 24, 659–686

Lovaas, O.I. (1981) *Teaching Developmentally Disabled Children: The Me Book*. Baltimore: University Park Press

Lovaas, O.I. (1987) Behavioural treatment and normal intellectual and educational functioning in autistic children. *Journal of Consulting and Clinical Psychology*, 55, 3–9

McEachin, J., Smith, T. and Lovaas, O. (1993) Long-term outcome for children with autism who received early intensive behavioural treatment. *American Journal of Mental Retardation*, 97 (4), 359–372

Mesibov, G. and Howley, M. (2003) *Accessing the Curriculum for Pupils with Autistic Spectrum Disorders*. London: David Fulton

Mesibov, G., Shea, V. and Schopler, E. (2004) *The TEACCH Approach to Autism Spectrum Disorders*. New York: Plenum Press

Morris, W. (2002) An examination of the National Autistic Society's EarlyBird Programme for parents of children with autistic spectrum disorders. *Good Autism Practice Journal. Early Intervention Edition*. Kidderminster: BILD

Myles, Brenda Smith (2001) *Asperger Syndrome and Adolescence: Practical Solutions for School Success*. London: Jessica Kingsley

Nally, B. (1999) *Austism and the Family – Reactions in Families*. London: National Antistic Society

National Initiative for Autism: Screening and Assessment (NIASA) (2003) *National Autism Plan for Children. NAP-C: Plan for the Identification, Assessment and Diagnosis of Children with ASDs*. London: National Autistic Society

Nind, M. and Hewett, D. (1994) *Access to Communication*. London: David Fulton

Parents and Professionals Autism (PAPA) Department of Education, Department of Education and Science, NI (2003) *Autistic Spectrum Disorder – A Teacher's Toolkit CD-ROM*

(2003) *Keyhole Autism Training Project*

(2006) *Rainbow Resource Kit* **www.autismni.org**

PEACH website **www.peach.org.uk/Home/**

Peeters, T. and Gillberg, C. (1999) *Autism: Medical and Educational Aspects*. London: Whurr

Plimley, L.A. and Bowen, M. (2006a) *Autistic Spectrum Disorders in the Secondary School*. London: Sage

Plimley, L.A. and Bowen, M. (2006b) *Supporting Pupils with Autistic Spectrum Disorders*. London: Sage

QCA/DfEE (2000) *Curriculum Guidance for the Foundation Stage*. London: QCA

Reed, P., Osborne, L. and Corness, M. (2006) Lecture given by Professor Phil Reed at the second International Autism Cymru conference. May 2006. Available at **www.awares. org**

Reed, P., Osborne, L. and Waddington, E.M.(2006) Lecture given by Professor Phil Reed at the second International Autism Cymru conference. May 2006. Available at **www.awares.org**

Robins, D.L., Fein, D., Barton, M.L and Green, J.A. (2001) The Modified Checklist for Autism in toddlers (M CHAT): An initial study investigating the early detection of autism and pervasive developmental disorders. *Journal of autism and developmental disorders, 31(2), 131–144*

Schopler, E. and Mesibov, G. (1995) Structured teaching in the TEACCH approach, in E. Schopler and G. Mesibov (eds) *Learning and Cognition in Autism*. New York: Plenum Press

Scott, F.J., Baron-Cohen, S., Bolton, P. and Brayne, C. (2002) The CAST (Childhood Asperger Syndrome Test) – Preliminary Development of a UK Screen for Mainstream Primary-School-Age Children. *Autism* 6(2), 9–31

Scottish CCC (1999) *Curriculum Framework for Children 3–5*. Dundee: Scottish Consultative Council on the Curriculum

Shea, V. (2004) A perspective on the research literature related to early intensive behavioural intervention for young children with autism. *Autism,* 8(4), 349–367

Shields, J. (1999) The NAS EarlyBird programme. Paper presented at Autism 99 internet conference

Shields, J. (2000) Preschool programmes, in A. Nye (ed.) *The Autism Handbook*. London: NAS

Siddles, R., Mills, R. and Collins, M. (1997) SPELL – The National Autistic Society approach to education. *Communication,* Spring 1997, 8–9

Smith, C. and McSpadden, L. (2002) Early interventions in autism: an LEA response. *Good Autism Practice Journal. Early Years edition*

Smith, P.G. (2005) A map for families with autistic children. *Early Education*, Spring 3–5

Sunderland University **http://osiris.sunderland.ac.uk/autism/**

Sussman, F. (1999) *More than Words*. Toronto: Hanen Centre

Walker-Jones, E. (2005). *My Brother Gwern.* Aberystwyth: Autism Cymru Publications

Wall, K. (2004) *Autism and Early Years Practice.* London: Paul Chapman

Waltz, M. (2005) *Metaphors of autism and autism as a metaphor.* **www.inter-disciplinary. net/mso/hid/hid2/hid03s11a.htm**

Wellman, J. (2005) Talk given to Prior's Court school on 6 July

Welsh Assembly Government (WAG) (2002) *The SEN Code of Practice for Wales*

Welsh Assembly Government (WAG) (2003a) *The Graduated Response:The Handbook of Good Practice*

Welsh Assembly Government (WAG) (2003b) *Statutory Assessments and Statements of Special Educational Need: The Handbook of Good Practice*

Welsh Assembly Government (WAG) (2006a) *Policy review of SEN. Part 2: Statutory Assessment framework (statementing)*

Welsh Assembly Government (WAG) (2006b) *Foundation Phase Pilot: First Year Evaluation Report*. Cardiff: National Assembly for Wales

Welsh Assembly Government (WAG) (2006c) *The Role of the Special Educational Needs Co-ordinator: The Handbook of Good Practice*

West Midlands Regional Partnership Project (2001) *Autistic Spectrum Disorders: A comprehensive report on the identification, training and provision, focusing on the needs of children and young people with an autistic spectrum disorder and their families in the West Midlands.* **www.westmidlandsrcp.org.uk**

Williams, D. (1996) *An Inside-Out Approach.* London Jessica Kingsley

Wing, L. (1988) The continuum of autistic characterisitics, in E. Schopler and G.B. Mesibov (eds) *Diagnosis and Assessment in Autism*. New York: Plenum Press

Wing, L. (1996) *The Autistic Spectrum*. London: Constable

Wing, L. and Gould, J. (1979) Severe impairments of social interaction and associated abnormalities in children: Epidemiology and classification. *Journal of Autism and Developmental Disorders, 9,* 11–29

Wing, L., Leekham, S. and Gould, J. (2002) The Diagnostic Interview for Social and Communication Disorders: background, inter-rater reliability and clinical use. *Journal of Child Psychology and Psychiatry 2002,* (43), 307–325

World Health Organisation (1993) *Mental disorders: A glossary and guide to their classification in accordance with the 10th revision of the International Classification of Diseases (ICD 10)*. Geneva: WHO

Useful websites

All websites checked 13/06/06

EARLYBIRD	**www.nas.org.uk** (keyword search EarlyBird)
GREENSPAN	**www.coping.org/earlyin/floortm.htm**
HANEN	**www.hanen.org**
INTENSIVE INTERACTION	**www.intensiveinteraction.co.uk**
LOVAAS	**www.lovaas.com**
NAS	**www.nas.org.uk**
OPTION	**www.option.org**
PECS	**www.pecs.org.uk**
(international site)	**www.pecs.com**
PORTAGE	**www.portage.org.uk**
SOCIAL STORIES	**www.thegraycenter.org**
SPELL	**www.nas.org.uk** (key word search SPELL)
TEACCH	**www.teacch.com**

Sources of information

ASD-specific organisations
Help is available at national, regional and local levels. Here are some useful organisations known to the authors.

National Autistic Society
393 City Rd
London
EC1V 1NE

Tel 020 7833 2299 for general enquiries
Helpline: 0845 070 4004
Parent to Parent support line: 0800 9 520 520
Email: **nas@nas.org.uk**
Website: **www.nas.org.uk**

Autism Northern Ireland (PAPA)
Donard
Knockbracken Healthcare Park
Saintfield
Belfast
BT8 8BH

Tel 0208 9040 1729
Email: **info@autismni.org**
Website: **www.autismni.org**

The Scottish Society for Autism
Head Office
Hilton House
Alloa Business Park
Whins Road
Alloa FK10 3SA

Tel 01259 720044
Email: **autism@autism-in-scotland.org.uk**
Website: **www.autism-in-scotland.org.uk**

Autism Cymru, Wales's national charity for autism
National Office
6 Great Darkgate St
Aberystwyth
Ceredigion
SY23 1DE

Tel 01970 625256
Email: **sue@autismcymru.org**
Website: **www.awares.org**

Education

For free copies of *The Special Educational Needs Code of Practice* and the useful booklet *Special Educational Needs (SEN): A Guide for Parents and Carers,* contact:

The Publications Department
The Department for Education and Skills
PO Box 5050
Sherwood Park
Annesley
Nottingham
NG15 ODJ

Tel 0845 6022260
Email: **dfes@prolog.uk.com**
Website: **www.dfes.gov.uk/sen**

IPSEA offers independent, free advice on the duties of local authorities regarding the educational needs of children with SEN:

Independent Panel for Special Educational Advice (IPSEA)
6 Carlow Mews
Woodbridge
Suffolk
IP12 1EA

Advice Line (England and Wales): 0800 018 4016
(Scotland): 0131 454 0082
(Northern Ireland): 01232 705654
Website: **www.ipsea.org.uk**

Centre for Studies on Inclusive Education (CSIE) – for information and advice on educating children with SEN in mainstream schools:
New Redland
Frenchay Campus
Coldharbour Lane
Bristol
BS16 1QU

Tel 0117 344 4007
Fax 0117 344 4005
Website: **www.inclusion.org.uk**

Financial

Disability Alliance campaigns for disabled people and their families and can offer benefits entitlement advice:
Universal House
88-94 Wentworth St
London
E1 7SA

Tel 020 7247 8776
Fax: 020 7247 8765
Website: **www.disabilityalliance.org**

Disability Benefit Enquiry Line: for benefits advice contact Freephone 0800 882200

Disability Living Allowance Advice Line: contact 08457 123456 (local rate)

Practical

RADAR campaigns and provides information on disability issues. RADAR keys unlock public toilets for the disabled and are a boon for parents out and about with an autistic child of the opposite gender from themselves:
12 City Forum
250 City Rd
London
EC1V 8AF

Tel 020 7250 3222
Fax: 020 7250 0212
Minicom: 020 7250 4119
Email: **radar@radar.org.uk**
Website: **www.mencap.org.uk**

Legal

The Children's Legal Centre
University of Essex
Wivenhoe Park
Colchester CO4 3FQ
An independent, national charity concerned with law and policy affecting children and young people. They operate an Education Law and Advocacy Unit and their lawyers and barristers provide free legal advice on all aspects of education law. Contact: 0845 120 2966 (charged at local rate) from 10am – 1pm

Glossary

ABA	Applied Behavioural Analysis
ACCAC	Qualifications, Curriculum and Assessment Authority for Wales
ADHD	Attention Deficit Hyperactivity Disorder
Aetiology	The root cause of a condition or disease
AS	Asperger syndrome
Autism Cymru	Wales's national charity for ASDs
CAMHS	Child and Adolescent Mental Health Services
CAST	Childhood Asperger Syndrome Test
CHAT	Checklist for Autism in Toddlers
Code of Practice	Guidance on the identification and assessment of pupils with SEN (England, Northern Ireland and Wales)
DENI	Department of Education Northern Ireland
DfES	Department for Education and Skills (England)

DIAGNOSTIC AND ASSESSMENT TOOLS	
ADI-R	Autism Diagnostic Interviews Revised (Lord et al., 1994)
ADOS	Autism Diagnostic Observation Schedule (Lord et al., 1989)
ASDI	Asperger Syndrome Diagnostic Interview (Gillberg et al., 2001)
DISCO	Diagnostic Interview for Social and Communication Disorders (Wing et al., 2002)
PL-ADOS	Prelinguistic Autism Diagnostic Observation Schedule (DiLavore et al., 1995)

DoH	Department of Health (England)
DSM IV	*Diagnostic and Statistical Manual* (Edition 4)
Early Bird Programme	Developed by the NAS and supports parents of young children with ASD post-diagnosis
Estyn	The inspection service in Wales
GAP	*Good Autism Practice* – a journal published by the British Institute of Learning Disabilities (BILD)
GP	General Practitioner
Graduated response	A staged approach to assessment of need used in England and Wales
Greenspan Floor Time	An interactive approach to ASD
Hanen Approach	Developed in Canada to increase functional communication
HMI	Her Majesty's Inspectors of Schools
IEP	Individual Education Programme
ICD 10	*International Classification of Diseases*
INSET	In-service training

Intensive Interaction	An interactive approach developed by Hewitt and Nind for individuals with SLD
LEA	Local Education Authority
M-CHAT	Modified Checklist for Autism in Toddlers
MMR	Measles, mumps, rubella triple vaccination
NAP-C	National Autism Plan for Children
NAS	National Autistic Society
NIASA	National Initiative for Autism: Screening and Assessment
NT	Neurotypical
Ofsted	A non-ministerial government body in England, responsible for the inspection of schools, LEAs, teacher-training institutions, youth work, colleges and early years provision
PAPA	Parents and Professionals for Autism/Autism Northern Ireland, the national charity for ASD in Northern Ireland
PCG	Primary care giver
PDD-NOS	Pervasive Developmental Disorder – Not Otherwise Specified
PECS	Picture Exchange Communication System
PHSE	Personal, social and health education
Portage	A programme developed to meet the needs of young children with SEN
PPS	Parent Partnership Services
School Fora	Developed by Autism Cymru to give teachers working with ASD in schools across Wales the opportunity to meet and exchange information
SEN	Special Educational Needs
SENCo	Special Educational Needs Co-ordinator
SENDA	The Special Educational Needs and Disability Act (2001)

SLD	Severe learning difficulties
SNAP Cymru	Special Needs Advisory Project in Wales
Social stories	A strategy developed by Carol Gray to teach individuals with ASD appropriate social skills
Son-Rise programme	A home-based programme developed in Massachusetts
SPELL	An acronym used to describe a learning environment that is Structured and Positive, shows Empathy, has an atmosphere of Low Arousal and has Links with parents
Statement of Special Educational Needs	A legal document that describes in detail a child's special educational needs and the range of provision that should be made available to meet those needs
TEACCH	Treatment and Education of Autistic and Communication handicapped Children
THOMAS approach	Developed in Hampshire, a programme that uses a range of strategies with a focus on the triad of impairments
Triad of impairments	Difficulties encountered by individuals with ASD in social understanding, social communication and rigidity of thought, noted by Lorna Wing
WAG	Welsh Assembly Government

Index

Added to the page number 'g' denotes the glossary and 't' denotes a table.